Breast Cancer Control

Breast Cancer Control

An Early Detection Programme

GISELA GÄSTRIN

M.D., Radiologist, B.Sc.
Health Education Consultant, Finland

ALMQVIST & WIKSELL INTERNATIONAL

STOCKHOLM · SWEDEN

ISBN 91-22-00438-6

Printed in Sweden by
Almqvist & Wiksell, Uppsala 1981

Contents

Preface

According to a conservative estimate, the number of breast cancers in the world female population approaches one million new cases every year. Many of these cases lead to premature deaths or a severe impairment of quality of life. The occurrence of these cancers cannot be prevented. But it has been proved that early treatment does increase survival and improve the women's quality of life compared to late treatment.

Today, early symptoms, such that are still not salient but quite well observable, often remain un-noticed because there is no search for them. Therefore many cases of breast cancer are detected and treated later than they could have been.

Consequently there is a possibility to attain a substantial saving of lives and human suffering if breast cancers could be detected and treated at an earlier stage than they usually are today.

The present book describes a programme aimed at achieving such early detection by establishing breast self-examination as a regular habit, practised in connection with a feed-back system and automatic referral to a breast specialist. Not only do its educational strategies guard against fear arousal. Its other advantages would also seem to be considerable. It minimizes delays on the part of patients and doctors alike. It can lessen the pressure of work on medical personnel. And it is inexpensive to implement.

It should be pointed out that a programme of this kind will be urgently needed also when mammography screening programmes are being in operation, since these can neither provide frequent enough examinations nor achieve a truly full geographical coverage of a whole nation.

The book gives an account of the larger context in which the programme was developed (Chapter I), it describes the programme principles (Chapter II) and a project in which the programme was finally tested (Chapter III). Implementation experiences are also reported (Chapter IV) and recommendations about how to keep the programme running are given (Appendix).

It should be noted that this new programme is not a new variety of screening programme. Instead it is a basically educational programme which can make use of existing public health care systems to involve virtually all women in a continuous activity. This feasability of a really large scale implementation stands out as one of the most innovative and important features of the programme.

Acknowledgements

I should like to thank the leaders and members of two Finnish women's organizations, Marttaliitto and Finlands Svenska Marthaförbund, for enabling me to carry out my project with 56 177 members; to my contact-person, Kaija Kauppinen, I owe thanks for her assistance with the field work. The Martha-organizations also brought the programme to the attention of The Associated Country Women of the World (ACWW) with the result that recommendations were adopted on a globale scale.

The Finnish Ministry of Health and National Board of Health, the medical association Finska Läkaresällskapet, the Signe and Ane Gyllenberg Foundation among others were interested in new ideas for the health-care of large groups of women, and awarded me fellowships for which I am grateful.

During the project stage I also received fellowships and assistance from the World Health Organization. For this I am grateful, and I should particularly like to thank Dr. Ramona Lunt of the WHO Cancer Unit.

For valuable co-operation during the evaluation stage of the project my thanks are due to The Finnish Cancer Registry.

For valuable co-operation and constructive criticism during the evaluation stage of the project my thanks are due to Dr. Patricia Hobbs, Project Chairman for Reports on Public Education about Cancer, UICC.

To Professor Pekka Virtama and Professor Carl-Erik Unnérus I would like to express my utmost appreciation for their expert advice and support, and I would like to thank my colleagues and the nurses, who through their devoted co-operation, made possible the success of this project. Also I extend my thanks to artist Henrik Tikkanen for his exquisite illustrations which women find som pleasing.

And lastly, I am deeply grateful to my children Jan Martin and Per Wilhelm, for all their practical help over the years, and for their patience.

Gisela Gästrin
Helsinki 1981

Chapter I

The fight against breast cancer – background situation

Epidemiological considerations

Between the various kinds of cancer there are differences in the nature of the illness, in the appropriate treatment, and in the response to be expected to treatment. Furthermore, the actual cause of the disease varies.

Certain types of cancer are linked to features of life-style. Smokers, for example, get smoker's lung cancer: non-smokers do not. For these types of cancer, the so-called primary prevention is possible; the cause can be entirely eliminated.

But primary prevention is not possible for breast cancer. There are many risk factors associated to breast cancer. It has long been known that there is a relation with the reproductive function: first menstruation at an early age, first pregnancy at a late age, menopause at a late age, nulliparity are all associated with enhanced risk. A relation has been shown with viruses, with injuries, with radiation and with certain breast diseases and history of familial breast cancer. But by far the greatest element of risk is related to age: the incidence of breast cancer rises after the age of 30 years, being greater with increasing age. The nature of the disease varies according to the patient's age (Clemmesen 1948).

One of the most important areas today for epidemiological research is diet. During recent years, studies have been made of the relation between breast cancer, estrogen metabolism and animal fat consumption. Preliminary results suggest that the mean plasma level of certain estrogen hormones is 50 % higher for omnivorous people than for vegetarians, a difference which could explain the relatively low incidence of breast cancer in vegetarian women (Adlercreutz et al. 1979). The geographical spread of breast cancer would thus be tidily accounted for; the disease is more frequent in highly developed countries, which consume more animal fat than poorer countries. After further research it may be possible to reduce some of the risks of breast cancer by means of dietary recommendations.

In the meantime, however, priority must clearly be given to so-called secondary prevention, which in this case means early diagnosis.

Incidence

The number of breast cancer cases registered is annually increasing. Two of the reasons for this are obvious: there have been improvements in diagnostics; and females born during the post-war period are now arriving at the vulnerable age.

The increase is highest in industrialized countries. In the United States one out of every 14 women is likely to develop the disease, and there are approximately 90000 new cases registered each year (Haskell et al. 1980). About 7 % of all women in industrialized countries will get breast cancer at some stage in their life (Shapiro et al. 1966, Stewens et al. 1969, Leis Jr 1970, Hinkamp 1971, De Saxe 1973, Lahti 1977). In poorer and developing countries, on the other hand, the incidence is markedly lower. National differences in breast cancer incidence can be seen in more detail from the following table:

BREAST CANCER INCIDENCE RATES PER 100000 WOMEN, AGE STANDARDIZED TO "WORLD POPULATION"
(from Cancer Incidence in Five Continents, vol. III, WHO, 1976)

CANADA		WEST GERMANY	
British Columbia	80.0	Saarland	50.6
Saskatchewan	62.8	ICELAND	49.5
U.S.A.		DENMARK	49.0
Connecticut	71.4	NORWAY	44.4
New York	57.2	BRAZIL	41.9
SWITZERLAND	70.6	GERMAN DEMOCRATIC REPUBLIC	33.4
ISRAEL		FINLAND	32.9
Europeans and Americans	60.8	SPAIN	30.6
Jews	55.5	YUGOSLAVIA	28.3
U.K.		INDIA	20.1
Birmingham	53.0	HUNGARY	19.8
SWEDEN	52.4	SINGAPORE	19.4
NEW ZEALAND	52.1	POLAND	18.5
		JAPAN	13.0

Mortality

Although there has been considerable increase in the number of registered breast cancer cases in most countries, breast cancer mortality has

BREAST CANCER DEATH RATES FOR DIFFERENT COUNTRIES
(1964–1965)
(from Clinical Oncology, UICC, Springer Verlag 1973)

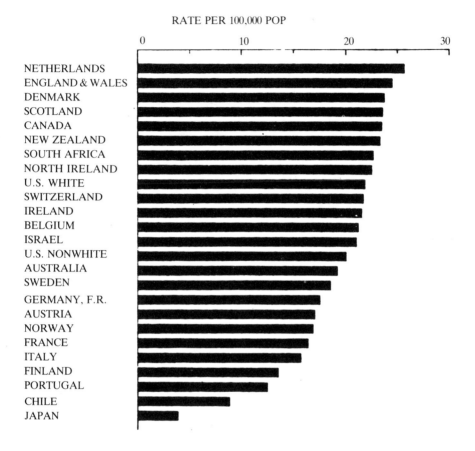

RATE PER 100,000 POP

declined over recent decades even if only very slightly and not in all countries. Various efforts towards achieving early diagnosis have not yet been shown to reduce breast cancer mortality. Mortality is still high world-wide. In countries with advanced medical treatment of breast cancer, about half the women die within five years after diagnosis. In countries with less advanced treatment the rates are even higher.

In the United States there are approximately 34 000 deaths caused by breast cancer each year (Haskell et al. 1980).

Clinical considerations

Effects of early detection

Clinical and histological staging of breast cancer has been made by different authors. In the following the 1978 figures of the clinical staging of the American Joint Committee, and the histologic staging of the National Surgical Adjuvant Breast project are presented.

SURVIVAL OF PATIENTS WITH BREAST CANCER RELATIVE TO CLINICAL AND HISTOLOGIC STAGE

	Crude Survival (%)	
	5 Yr	10 Yr
Clinical Staging		
Stage I		
Tumor <2 cm in diameter	85	
Nodes, if present, not felt to contain metastases		
Without distant metastases		
Stage II		
Tumors <5 cm in diameter	66	
Nodes, if palpable, not fixed		
Without distant metastases		
Stage III		
Tumor >5 cm or,	41	
Tumor any size with invasion of skin or attached to chest wall		
Nodes in supraclavicular area		
Without distant metastases		
Stage IV		
With distant metastases	10	
Histologic Staging:		
All patients	63.5	45.9
Negative axillary lymph nodes	78.1	64.9
Positive axillary lymph nodes	46.5	24.9
1–3 positive axillary lymph nodes	62.2	37.5
>4 positive axillary lymph nodes	32.0	13.4

According to this classification stage I cases are "early" ones, the tumour being less than 2 cm in diameter and there are negative axillary lymph nodes.

SURVIVAL: Patients with stage I breast cancers have the best prognosis while those with stage IV have the worst prognosis. But histopathologic examination of lymph nodes removed during mastectomy provides more precise prognostic information.

Prognosis worsens with each additional positive node found, patients with four or more positive nodes appear to have a much worse prognosis than either those with no positive nodes or those with one to three positive nodes (Henderson et al. 1980).

A well known study which is performed in England shows age corrected survival rates for women treated for breast cancers of different size. Where the tumour was 1 cm in diameter and there were negative axillary lymph nodes, about 80 % of the patients survived for twenty years after treatment. But there was still a higher death rate 20 years after primary treatment than in the age-matched normal population. Patients with tumours of 2 cm in diameter had lower survival rates and patients suffering from breast cancer tumours over 3 cm in diameter showed a rapid fall in survival within the first 5 years after treatment to about 60 %.

AGE-CORRECTED SURVIVAL RATES FOR WOMEN TREATED FOR BREAST CANCERS UP TO 3.0 CM IN DIAMETER (Duncan et al. 1976)

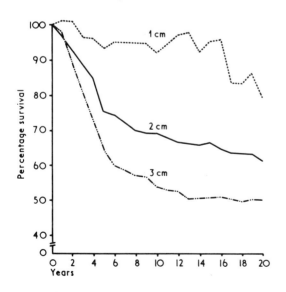

QUALITY OF LIFE: For patients who present themselves with small breast tumours and negative axillary lymph nodes there has been a shift from radical mastectomy towards less incapacitating surgery, being curative in proportion of cases. Already 40 years ago in Finland good results were obtained by treating early breast cancer tumours with local resection combined with radiotherapy (Mustakallio 1972). Today less incapacitating surgery such as simple mastectomy, subcutaneous mastectomy and tumour resection are commonly used where possible. These operations are in a number of cases complemented with plastic surgery, reconstruction of the breast, subcutaneous prostheses, etc. The use of surgery that is less incapacitating and has better cosmetic effect from the patient's point of view causes less physical and psychological incapacity to the woman. The factor which most influences prognosis is not the type of surgery performed but the extent of spread of the cancer at the time of treatment (Chamberlain 1978). This supports the idea that breast cancers should be detected as early as possible and thus limited surgery could be offered to the patients.

Tumour growth and detectability

Breast cancer varies enormously in its growth rates. The time required for beast cancer tumours to double in volume varies from about 100 to 1 000 days (Collins et al. 1979). If a tumour doubles in size every 100 days the time required for a single malignant cell to grow to a clinically detectable tumour of 1 cm in diameter would be about 8 years (Henderson et al. 1980). According to many authors there is diminished growth rate with increasing tumour size.

Breast cancer spreads from one or several focuses in the breast to regional lymph nodes if the primary tumour is not removed early. The dissemination to different organs can occur within a short or long time; the quantitative time required for spreading is not presently known.

The smallest lump detected by mammography examination in asymptomatic women has been described as 2 mm in diameter and the smallest lump found by women themselves by *accidental* observation was 2 cm in diameter (Ackerman 1979). The smallest lump found by active, *systematic* self-examination was according to experience by the present author 1 cm and by Canadian experience 0.5 cm in diameter (Wallace 1979). It should be kept in mind that the lump that is felt by palpation consists of both the tumour and of surrounding connective tissue. The size of the lump is therefore bigger than that of the tumour.

TUMOUR GROWTH AND DETECTABILITY IN BREAST CANCER

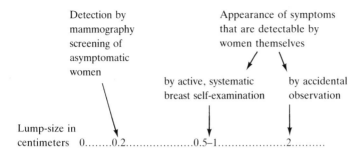

Since detection by systematic self-examination can occur at a substantially more early stage of tumour growth than by accidental observation, it is urgent to distinguish between these two categories.

The variation in growth rate and time-point for dissemination of breast cancer as well as women's own ability to detect symptoms calls for a multitude of measures to detect breast cancer cases at the earliest possible stage. But it must be remembered that lumps are by no means the only signs of breast cancer. All physicians know that there are other breast cancer symptoms too, most of them detectable by the women themselves. Some of these symptoms are seen by visual inspection and others are detectable by palpation.

The signs of breast cancer can be straightforward, and are thus easily noticible. According to the experience of the present author breast cancers that have been detected by self-examination where attention has been drawn to retraction of the nipple or the skin, bloody discharge from the nipple, have often turned out to be minimal infiltrating cancers less than 1 cm in diameter, in situ lobular cancers or even intraductal cancers. Only very seldom can a woman detect breast cancer by noticing enlarged lymph nodes in her axilla as a first breast cancer symptom; many people have enlarged nodes in the axilla without having breast cancer.

Every woman can learn to know what is normal for HER. Then she will be able to recognize changes from what is normal. This requires something more than accidental observation. It even requires more than sporadic self-examination; there is a need for systematic, regular self-examination.

Symptoms that women are able to detect in their breasts are as follows (Alcoe et al. 1979):

NON MALIGNANT CHANGES:
- One breast is slightly larger than the other
- Tenderness in the breasts beginning shortly before a menstrual monthly period and disappearing after the period is under way or finished
- Darkening of the nipples and areola with each pregnancy
- Redness from exposure to sun
- Increase in size of both breasts with weight gain

MALIGNANT CHANGES:
- Pain (infrequent in young women; frequent in older women)
- Unequal elevation of a breast
- Increase or decrease in size of a breast
- Retraction of the skin of the breast
- Orange coloured skin of the breast
- Assymetry of the nipples
- Retraction of the nipple
- The nipple is sore
- Bloody discharge from the nipple
- Hard lump or mass in the breast (one or both)

Procedures for detection

Accidental observation

About 90 % of the symptoms of breast cancer mentioned above are first detected by women themselves more or less by coincidence. And even if a woman detects breast cancer symptoms, she will not necessarily make an immediate appointment with a physician.

By the time the symptoms are examined by a physician, the average size of the breast cancer tumour is already 3.5 cm in diameter, and in many cases there is already some axillary spread – American investigators have found such spread in about 65 % of all cases during the 1960's and in about 50 % during the 1970's (Gershon-Cohen 1967, Aarts 1969). For those women who, after observation of symptoms as mentioned above, come to a medical examination, mammography, as well as mammography in combination with cytology, gives a correct diagnosis in about 95 % (Standerskiöld-Nordenstam et al. 1980, Hillerdal 1979). Even more effectively mammography can be complemented with stereotactic needle biopsy, as in a Swedish study (Nordenström 1979).

Sometimes breast cancer symptoms in young women are detected by visual inspection or palpation by the women themselves or by medical personnel before they can be detected by mammography and other techniques. On the other hand mammography will occasionally reveal a cancer, that cannot be revealed by other clinical examination techniques (Lesnick 1977).

A study in Australia in 1970 indicated that only 24 % of the women diagnosed as new breast cancer cases presented their symptoms within a month of finding them, and that in at least a third of the new cases in 1974 there was a delay of three or more months. Later studies indicate that 40 % had shown up within three months after accidental observation of symptoms (Hill et al. 1977). This "patients delay" has been reported to be the result of anxiety as late as in 1974 (Selvini 1974). Since then quite new potentialities of breast self-examination have been reported.

But even if a woman does report to a physician immediately after self-detection of symptoms there can also be "doctor's delay". 18 % of the breast cancer patients in a Swedish study group, on reporting their symptoms, failed to receive a quick diagnosis. The delay ranged from two weeks to four and a half years (Arner et al. 1978). Physicians, then as well, can hesitate or feel unsure, even if women demonstrate symptoms which are typical for breast cancer and which they themselves know about. Sometimes cooperation between one specialist and another does not run smoothly.

Most women do not know of a specialist to whom they can turn. They report to their family doctor or gynaecologist, who, instead of referring every case to an experienced surgeon, radiologist or oncologist, sometimes hesitates or gives a negative diagnosis. Roughly 15 % of all breast cancer cases come to light as the result of the tumour's rapid growth after an initially negative clinical diagnosis (Strax 1977).

Sometimes it is a physician, and not the woman herself, who first detects a breast cancer, during a medical check-up or some screening process which is not aimed at the detection of breast cancer. But this too occurs in what can only be regarded as a somewhat accidental fashion and the woman may acquire a false sense of security from one such examination to the next.

But clearly, in the absence of a more comprehensive system the efforts of physicians and nurses should by no means be undervalued. Many gynaecologists are already uniting with surgeons and radiologists in breast cancer detection.

21

Systematic detection

Some background viewpoints

Since breast cancer can develop so rapidly, the only way in which it can be satisfactorily detected is by frequent and systematic examination. This can be performed either by medical personnel or by the women themselves. In either case, suspect breast cancer symptoms should then be immediately referred to an experienced surgeon working in co-operation with radiologists, cytologists, oncologists and pathologists.

So far, however, no entire female population has had either a systematic search for symptoms or a system of automatic referral to a breast specialist for symptoms detected. What is needed are permanent programmes with a spread that is geographically complete.

In 1974 the Council of Europe established three criteria for diseases that can and should be diagnosed through systematic search programmes:

1. The disease is an obvious burden for the individual and/or the community in terms of suffering of economic and social costs.
2. The disease goes through an initial latent stage during which it can be detected by appropriate tests.
3. Treatment is available which has been shown to improve the prognosis for the disease.

Breast cancer obviously fulfils the first criterion. Breast cancer is still a physical and psychological burden for every individual who gets the disease and has to undergo difficult treatment because of late diagnosis. Breast cancer causes enormous economic and social costs to the community because of the need for expensive treatment and rehabilitation in late coming patients and because there are cost contributions to the national production due to lenghty sick-leave from work and premature deaths.

Breast cancer fulfils the second criterion too, since various diagnostic techniques and certain screening programmes have shown that the time involved for breast cancer to develop where it can be detected can be shortend.

The third criterion is also satisfied, thanks to the good prognosis for those who are treated early, especially in the light of surgery, radiation and other treatment methods that have been developed and that are less incapacitating, opening the way for better quality of life.

We are now going to look at the two main procedures for systematic detection, screening and breast self-examination.

Screening procedures

The benefits of screenings for cervical cancer have raised the question about the benefits of screenings for early detection of breast cancer as well.

So far the most well known screening programme is the one used in the study of the Health Insurance Plan of Greater New York, The HIP study. It began in 1964 and examined the effects of annual physical examinations and mammography examination on a study group of about 30 000 women and a control group of the same size. A statistically significant difference in survival was found in women over 50 years only, and their breast cancer mortality was reduced by at least one-third and there has been a persistence of breast cancer mortality reduction over a twelve year period. Mammography-detected breast cancers were extremely early cases, often cured, with a survival rate of 78 % for ten years. The physical examination alone has been credited with about 70 % of the benefit of the HIP study (Strax 1980). Soon after the early results on mortality became available from the HIP study an extensive Breast Cancer Detection Demonstration Project (BCDDP) was started in 1973 under the sponsorship and support of the National Cancer Institute (USA) and American Cancer Society. A quarter of a million women from 35 to 74 years of age were enrolled in this project in 27 screening centres for a cycle of 5 annual screenings with mammography, physical examination of the breasts and thermography. Provision was made for a Data Management Center to collect data on the results of the screening examinations, biopsy findings, and personal background information from the screened women. In this study a great amount of the new breast cancers found were so-called minimal cancers. Again the results do actually provide an indication of the benefits for women over 50 (Shapiro 1978).

The possible risks of mammography, have been discussed by other experts, for instance at a conference arranged by the American Cancer Society in 1979.

One speaker stated: It has been suggested that only slowly growing carcinomas are discovered in the preinvasive stage and that screening for early detection is, therefore, of little value. More aggressive neoplasms, it is postulated, are capable of passing through all stages of the natural history between screening examinations. Analysis of data from the BCDDP should confirm or refuse this hypothesis (Gallager 1979).

Another speaker stated: It is likely that the breast is the organ most sensitive to radiation carcinogenesis in post-pubertal women. Studies of different exposed populations have yielded remarkably consistent re-

23

sults, in spite of wide differences in underlying breast cancer rates and conditions of exposure. Excess risk is approximately proportional to dose, and relatively independent of ionization density and fractionization of dose (Land 1979).

Elsewhere, another expert has stated that routine annual mammography should be restricted to women with a previous history of breast cancer; evidence about the optimal frequency for universal screening has not yet been brought together (Croll 1977). Even for wealthy countries the cost is quite prohibitive, and the personnel is just not available (Beard 1966). Some Swedish experts, on the other hand, judge that the technique's advantages outweigh the risks; moreover, they have developed a technique using only small radiation doses (Lundgren 1980).

Research in screening for breast cancer and experiences from different breast cancer screening programmes have shown that early detection of breast cancer is possible in screened groups of women and that this does influence life expectancy and quality of life in women who are offered those screenings (Andersson 1980). However, breast cancer is not always detectable by mammography technique in women under 50 years of age. And in many cases of breast cancer the screening interval of one year is even too long: There will be many women who are not summoned to screening at timepoints that are ideal from the point of view of the occurence of the individual woman's breast cancer. Therefore, only a minimal fraction of the women in the world can be offered high quality and safe screenings often enough. And there is in all screenings a group of non-respondents.

But, mammography examination, as well as examination with other technical equipment can provide diagnosis in a way that is both specific and sensitive to old and young women when they have already found symptoms themselves and show up for examination. The skill of the women to detect breast cancer symptoms should be used in a more systematic and effective way and measures should be provided to direct the woman to show up at a specific physician's office if she detects symptoms. The sensitivity of annual screenings should be compared with the benefits of high frequency offered by other methods. The hope has been focused on programmes of health education (Bailar 1976, Räf 1979).

Breast self-examination (BSE)

The idea of breast self-examination immediately raises four questions.
First, can women really detect breast cancer symptoms themselves? It

24

has been shown in most countries that women themselves are able to detect both non-malignant and malignant changes in their own breasts. The breast cancer symptoms can be observed by inspection and palpation. A woman's own ability to detect symptoms in her own breasts is often greater than that of a physician who is not a breast cancer expert. There are many examples of women who show up with symptoms that they have detected, but physicians do sometimes ignore such information and they must later admit that they were wrong in doing so (author's experience).

Secondly, how often should BSE be practised? The time in which a breast cancer increases in size varies from case to case. The growth to self-detectable size may take place very rapidly. Optimal conditions for inspection and palpation by physicians and the women themselves prevail after menstruation, when the breasts are soft and not tender to touch. It is generally agreed that BSE should therefore be carried out on a regular monthly basis – even by women who for various reasons have no menstruations.

Thirdly, how should BSE be carried out? A detailed description will be given in "Appendix". Perhaps the most important points is that the BSE technique used should be a combination of visual inspection and cautious palpation. The cautiousness is of utmost importance since some experts believe that injuries to the breasts can actually be one of the causes of breast cancer (Koulumies 1956).

Lastly, how can women be really motivated to practise BSE on a regular monthly basis? This is the greatest problem and the communication methods so far adopted have varied very much from programme to programme as will be illustrated below.

At certain instances BSE is brought about as a secondary component of a screening programme, both screenings for breast cancer and screenings for cervical cancer or other health counseling.

At first sight it might look like an efficient system to have BSE instruction attached to screenings. Although, representing a step forward, there are very serious weaknesses in this method. One is coverage. Nowhere have screenings been offered to every woman in a nationwide population and very seldom on a continuous basis. Furthermore the coverage is still more reduced by non-respondents among those to which screenings have actually been offered. Another weakness has usually been the lack of continued surveillance and frequently enough repeated encouragement of BSE in these connections. A conclusion of the above observations would be that there is need for programmes where BSE is given the role as the primary component of the programme.

There have also been health education projects consisting in dissemination of BSE instruction where, consequently, BSE is given a primary role. The comprehensiveness of such programmes has varied immensely. Some "programmes" consist of nothing else than making a pamphlet available to "the large public". Today, this is quite obviously not enough.

There have also been examples of programmes using other media.

In Denmark during the 1950's and in Australia during the 1960's, there were television campaigns continuously urging women to practise regular BSE and report symptoms to a medical centre. A similar campaign, (designed by the present author), was run in Finland in connection with the project to be described later in this book. In every case there was an increase in the number of women reporting with symptoms, but this tailed off as soon as the television transmissions came to an end.

In British Columbia the delay in diagnosis and long term survival in breast cancer has been followed from 1945 to 1975 in a programme based on mass communication. "Public education" was pursued since 1938 and since 1956 films about BSE were used.

National surveys in Canada have reported that the proportion of women stating that they regularly examine their breasts rose from 20 % in 1960 to 63 % in 1975 and that those using breast self-examination have shorter delay times. Long term survival was greater in patients with a shorter delay between the appearance of self-detectable symptoms and clinical diagnosis made by physicians (Elwood et al. 1980).

The aspects of the acceptance of breast self-examination have been studied at the University Hospital of South Manchester in England.

As part of a large-scale study of the teaching of breast self-examination to women in the general population such factors have been investigated that affect acceptance of the idea and the regular practice of BSE. It has further been investigated whether such health education might have an influence on women's anxiety and concern about breast cancer and their own vulnerability. Around 700 women from existing women's groups were taught BSE in 1979. The study results reflect the women's degree of awareness of BSE. Pre-teaching questionaires were used and the study excluded information about the performance of BSE. Women's awareness of BSE is related to their opinions regarding breast cancer in three important areas:

Women with a high awareness of BSE
– are worried about getting cancer

26

- are more confident about the possibility of detecting cancer at an early stage
- are more optimistic about the chance of curing breast cancer detected early.

Women who were examiners at the time of attending the information meetings were
- more optimistic in their opinions concerning early detection and the curability of breast cancer
- more concerned about the possibility that they themselves might get cancer.

It was found that only 15 % of the women studied at the pre-teaching stage were "very worried". Women who develop this concern may actively seek to be taught BSE, or may be more receptive to health education related to breast cancer. The concern motivates women towards BSE (Hobbs et al. 1980).

Practically all BSE programmes to date could be described as "one-dimensional", most of them being mainly oriented towards teaching BSE.

However, as previously mentioned, there are numerous dimensions of the problem situation that need being attended to. What deserves attention are further aspects of the acceptance of breast self-examination by the individual woman, her compliance with BSE, a check on the regularity in her BSE and a referral system to a breast cancer specialist for the individual women who detect symptoms.

A multidimensional programme that takes all these aspects into account will be described in the following chapters of this book. In this programme educational aspects will play a dominating role. Therefore, before describing the new programme and the project in which it is tested we should have a background overview of the different communication aspects regarding breast cancer and breast self-examination.

Communication aspects

Mass communication

General information about breast cancer can have some effect on breast cancer detection, sometimes a beneficial effect and sometimes not. Mass communication can convey information and increase knowledge and it can to some extent shape attitudes, but it can hardly influence behaviour and instil a suitable habit of life-long personal health care (James 1974).

Non health education oriented mass communication has now reached a very high level of technical expertise and equipment. Much professionalism goes into the presentation of the message in radio, TV and the press. The impact is sometimes enormous and the audience huge. But none of this guarantees the quality of the actual message itself. And cancer is still surrounded by so much sensationalism, so much playing on people's deepest fears, that more factual, reassuring information about breast cancer and BSE can easily pass unnoticed.

The myth about the incurability of cancer is at least fifty years old and as strong as ever. Based on ignorance or inaccurate and out-of-date information, it makes people frightened and apathetic. It may make some women perform BSE and report a breast cancer symptom. But it makes also many hesitate to do so.

It is quite pointless to adopt a sensationalistic approach, or to try and frighten women into action. Regrettably, even some health-educators speak of what they are doing as "propaganda", an attitude which is entirely counterproductive.

Many women are powerfully influenced by the world of fashion and by what one might call the cult of the bosom. Psychologists have shown, too, that women are led to feel that their breasts are intimately associated with their very identity as women. So the threat of breast cancer comes to seem especially insidious.

For all this, however, the mass media has also adopted a more constructive approach. An excellent example has been the news items about the wives of prominent American politicans. Through the mass media these admirable women stimulated millions of others to practice BSE, and gave thousands of other patients new hope of a cure. They showed that breast cancer need not entail anxiety, suffering and death. And the personal touch they gave this message resulted in a wide-spread change in women's attitudes.

No other branch of medicine has been so thoroughly investigated as cancer – its causes, its growth, its prognosis – and our understanding of breast cancer in particular has made great strides. The time for myths is past, and a woman detecting symptoms herself is entitled to a certain degree of confidence. But neither the mass media nor the medical profession itself has done enough to spread the good news. Although information of a more factual nature is readily available in medical journals, it does not yet compete with more sensationalistic accounts. Physicians and nurses have known for many years that breast cancer is no longer the problem it used to be. They know: that early diagnosis is possible; that surgery nowadays is often much less radical and incapacitating than it used to be; and that even difficult cases will respond to repeated radiation.

Health education that consists of mass communication is the type of communication most often used by cancer societies, health authorities, etc. for informing women about the need for regular BSE. And messages planned with medical and health education expertise do stand some chance of influencing both knowledge and attitudes.

Health education oriented information through mass communication channels has sometimes consisted of the mere distribution of brochures, which has turned out to be unsatisfactory. Such efforts have often served to make women passive and frightened. Sometimes, one message will seem to contradict another, and particularly as regards the technique of breast self-examination. Some brochures recommend the cautious approach. Others recommend massage or finger-tip palpation. This sows the seeds of doubt: "The experts themselves are not sure what they mean".

Often, too, the message concentrates only on BSE itself, finishing simply with a curt piece of advice: "If you find any symptoms get in touch with a doctor". This gives only a very general guideline. It does not, so to speak, take the woman into its care. It is not personal and reassuring. She finds the responsibility for BSE placed firmly on her own shoulders, yet receives no real encouragement to do anything about it. What is needed, clearly, is some check on her acceptance of the message. One must positively find out whether she carries out BSE regularly. One must do everything to maximize the likelihood that she will report any symptoms. And she herself must confidently know that there is some such system geared to her personal well-being. After all, from her point of view a mass communication message is nothing more than a sporadic and one-way event. A message continuously sent, whether through the press, TV or radio, or in brochures, is not continuously received; it must compete, too, with all the other messages to which a woman is daily exposed.

On the few occasions when the message got through to the woman and made some impression, she had no opportunity to ask questions and start a dialogue. Thus it may well have created a counter-productive misunderstanding and anxiety.

To return to the point made earlier, the persuasiveness of health education by mass communication is dependent on the degree to which it gives the individuals of the target group a sense of security. But person-to-person communication has, as already pointed out, a greater influence than mass communication on people's health behaviour.

Person-to-person communication

Personal communication not in the form of organized health education often takes place as conversations between women in various groupings and situations, with healthy women, potential breast cancer patients and confirmed patients all taking part. Most often, perhaps, breast cancer problems are discussed in hospitals, between one patient and another or between women and the nursing staff. Many women do not realize that, although there was a time when treatment used to be the same for all patients, nowadays it can vary much, depending on how soon the disease is diagnosed. Women try to explain the variations in their own way, and this is where one communicant can easily influence another. Both between individuals and in groups, a general feeling of either fear or security can result from the articulacy of a single strong personality. People sometimes express themselves very emphatically when they actually know very little. Perhaps medically trained personnel should discuss things with their patients more.

Personal communication between women generally tends to instil fear rather than hope. Yet it can also be very reassuring to hear of another woman's favourable experiences of the disease and its treatment. Women who come to learn of the disease in this way react more calmly if they get it themselves, as do physicians and nurses.

Health education that consists of person-to-person communication is more powerful than mass communication in influencing attitudes and health behaviour. It conveys information and advice on a personal basis, and allows questions to be asked. It can therefore rouse interest in BSE and help to establish it as a regular and lifelong habit. And this personalized and sympathetic approach is specially reassuring when exact information on BSE and symptom referral is received from a trustworthy person with special training in the field.

However, person-to-person communication, no matter how it is organized in practice, can be just as sporadic in effect as mass communication. Physicians and nurses may systematically teach BSE to every woman they meet, but every woman will not systematically learn or be motivated to perform BSE as a life-long habit. Just as when she reads brochures, a woman may acquire the knowledge without the habit. The present author has seen all too many instances of this in women urged to BSE during e.g. screenings for cervical cancer.

The reason for such negative outcome of an undoubtedly positive effort would most probably be two-fold. From the receiver's point of view it seems to be a sporadic, infrequent influence and, from the sender's point of view, it is a secondary kind of duty in relation to the primary components of screenings, breast consultations and other consultations. But other experiences are positive. E.g. in smoking cessation programmes it has been demonstrated that educational efforts of person-to-person type have been successful in providing changes in health behaviour even at a sporadic basis by first increasing motivation (Gästrin et al. 1975).

One more example is the following. In connection with special rehabilitation programmes for cancer patients, American breast cancer patients have for many years been the target of person-to-person communication. Their feelings about the disease are consequently more optimistic than those of, say, Swedish patients (The Gallup Organization 1976, Gyllensköld 1976). These efforts, pioneered by the American Cancer Society, have sometimes taken the form of visits by former patients to patients about to be operated on. There are also Therese Lasser's "Reach to Recovery" programme, aimed at rehabilitation, and Ella Bernhardt's more specific scheme for improving the individual fitting of prostheses.

In every case the reassuring message has largely been passed on by volunteer workers. No official organization can have a paid staff big enough to cope, and voluntary contacts have actually proved themselves very effective. In an operation of this size, no single volunteer is called upon to do more than she can, yet there is always *somebody* available when the need arises. The volunteer is there to help her fellow-woman at a crucial point. And with the return to normal life, the degree of help gradually lessens.

In 1970 the present author initiated a similar scheme in Finland, by initiating a cancer patient association to promote the medical, psychological and social adjustment of cancer patients, and of breast cancer patients in particular.

Education about BSE in order to detect breast cancer symptoms through BSE, however, differs in aim from communication in connection with rehabilitation. The need for the person-to-person contact, and for the active attention of they key-person, does not gradually diminish, as is

31

the case in rehabilitation. Support is needed constantly if BSE is to become the life-long habit it should be.

This is a reason why the key-person should be recruited on something other than a voluntary basis. And since no single organization is likely to have enough qualified people, the existing public health services would seem to be the natural pool from which they could be drawn, when it comes to carry through a nationwide program.

The challenge

It has been shown by Duncan et al. that breast cancer patients with small tumours have a longer survival than those with large tumours. It has been shown by Mustakallio and others that limited surgery and reconstruction of the breast can be used in early detected breast cancer cases. For the individual patient treatment of early detected breast cancer means a quality of life that is considerably better than was earlier thought possible. Universal, sufficient and inexpensive screening is not available for all women in the world who need it. But research into breast cancer screening does show that *something* can be done to achieve early diagnosis.

Seen as a public health problem involving a large risk population, breast cancer calls for a variety of control measures. Screening programmes, programmes based on breast physical examination, and other efforts aimed at early diagnosis, BSE-centered programmes for example, can be launched side by side with programmes already in function offering a complete geographical coverage and short intervals between the control of individual women's breasts. It is the responsibility of decision makers to recommend and implement, and of physicians and other medical personnel to plan and supervise universal, frequent and inexpensive programmes aimed at catching detectable but still unnoticed cases, and cases of breast cancer which women know about but have not referred to a physician. Programmes for regular BSE and self-detection of symptoms have to be of highest quality.

The ability of women to detect different breast cancer symptoms themselves must be taken advantage of. Women should be motivated to practise monthly BSE as a life-long habit, unnecessary fears should be alleyed and women should be encouraged to consult a breast specialist without delay, if needed. BSE must be carried out in a cautious manner that is completely harmless for the individual woman. Continuous breast self-examination and, for symptomatic women, immediate contact with a breast specialist, should be built into a systematic programme just as breast physical examination or mammography are built into systematic screening programmes for asymptomatic women.

The target for a continuous breast self-examination programme should be

- All women over 20 who are not offered breast cancer screenings (in order to catch self-detectable cases)
- All women who are offered breast cancer screenings with annual intervals (in order to catch self-detectable "interval cancer cases").

The present chapter can perhaps best conclude by enforcing this impression with citations of some leading authorities in the field of health education:

"Too much health education is still conducted on no sort of scientific basis. Often it seems to spring from a vague but powerful feeling that something ought to be done about some serious current problem, such as needless deaths from cancer. Health education of this kind may sometimes be useful, but all too frequently it seems to satisfy the needs of the organizers to do *something*, rather than those of the community it is supposed to serve. There are limits to what can be done, whether by a large national organization or from local resources. But some form of evaluation of what is being done is needed, it we really want to know whether our resources are being deployed to the best advantage and whether we are achieving the objectives that were defined or would have been defined at the planning stage of the educational programme. This is the point of a major importance: for true evaluation to be possible, every public education programme must have declared objectives before it begins. Otherwise, honest measuring, or evaluating, can be relatively crude, say, by a simple count of those who do what is advised. Sometimes more sophisticated methods or interviewing truly representative sample of the population are needed. All may be effective in a given situation" (Wakefield 1974).

"Before entering into any concrete stage of planning in the field of preventive medicine, it will be necessary to visualize the mental situation of the potential target group of patients, and to analyze as closely as possible the aspects of the situation resulting from the projected preventive care operation, basing on the patient's viewpoint. ... All activities in the field of preventive medicine should be well prepared in a manner which should be specific for the relevant target groups" (Verres 1978).

In a Cancer Society Monograph in 1958, Haagensen said, "It is probable that, from the point of view of the greatest possible gain in early diagnosis, teaching women how to examine their own breasts is more important than teaching the technique of breast examinations to physicians, for we must keeep in mind the fact that at least 98 percent of the women who develop breast carcinoma discover their tumours themselves." Unfortunately, this is still true today. There is urgent need to focus research on methods to detect breast cancer in its early stages. "Caution is emphasized in widespread advocacy of breast self-examination without adequate supporting evidence of its efficacy. There is need for well designed prospective study of breast self-examination with full attention to a rigorous design and methodology." (Venet 1979).

The World Health Organization's Regional Office for Europe has in 1977 proposed as some of the major issues in cancer control: the planning and organization of services; training and evaluation, and the use of evaluation results; the implementation of existing knowledge; primary prevention and health education; secondary prevention and early detection.

An important step towards such an implementation consists in the working out of recommendations by authorative public health agencies. An example of such a set of recommendations is a 1980 report from the American Cancer Society on guidelines for cancer checkups. With regard to breast cancer this report says:

 • All women over 20 perform breast self-examination monthly. From 20 to 40 they should have a breast physical examination every three years. Those over 40 should have a breast physical examination every year.

  • Between 35 and 40, every woman ought to have a baseline mammogram as a point of reference. Women 40 to 49 should consult their physicians about their need for mammography.

 • Women over 50 should have a mammogram every year.

As a summary comment to the ACS recommendation the present author would like to point out that BSE is given the definitely basic and primary role. BSE is the only procedure that is being recommended for frequent continued, life-long practice already from the age of 20. The other procedures that are recommended to be introduced are serving as supplements but do never replace BSE or take over the role of BSE as the basic procedure.

The construction and publishing of this type of recommendation is a very important, but not the final step towards such large-scale, continued action which would constitute the implementation of the ideas of the recommendations. The need exists for a programme for action.

In conclusion the following can be said about BSE and self detection of breast cancer symptoms: BSE should be a primary and basic programme in the fight against breast cancer when it comes to large, nationwide programmes. But isolated teaching of BSE does not constitute a comprehensive programme which would make BSE a life-long, continuous and regular habit for every woman. It is SPORADIC in nature and it does not automatically refer a woman, who detects breast cancer symptoms herself, to a breast specialist, who offers the final diagnosis.

A step further (complementing screening programmes, breast physical examination and teaching BSE) one could speak of a "new dimension" in an entire programme in the fight against breast cancer: SYSTEMATIC BREAST SELF-EXAMINATION. And in order to achieve a systematic, life-long breast self-examination, a health education programme is needed that complements shortcomings in existing health education for early self-detection of breast cancer symptoms.

In the next chapter there will be a discussion about modelling a programme that could meet the requirements that have just been mentioned.

Chapter II

Modelling the programme for breast cancer control

Fundamental considerations

Until today different activities in order to achieve early diagnosis of breast cancer have been developed by medical and technical staff (e.g. medical examination with mammography and other equipment), by decision makers (e.g. arranging for screening programmes), and by health education staff (for motivating women to regular BSE).

From the individual woman's point of view the different activities offered do not constitute a comprehensive, geographically complete and continuous programme for breast cancer control. There is a need for further development not only what comes to medical technique or the administration of screening procedures, but also for developing health education procedures, in order to activate women to perform regular, correct BSE throughout their lives, to recognize breast cancer symptoms and to contact a breast specialist immediately if symtoms of breast cancer occur.

Many authors continue with the development of medical-technique for breast cancer diagnosis, others are arranging for screening administration procedures. The author of this present book deals with the development of health education, with special interest focused upon the situation from the woman's point of view.

Breast Cancer Control from the individual woman's point of view

SCREENING with mammography and/or other methods:
- not geographically complete
- not continuous and/or frequent enough
  (causes a false feeling of security)

BREAST PHYSICAL EXAMINATION by medical staff:
- not geographically complete
- not continuous and/or frequent enough
  (causes a false feeling of security)

BREAST SELF-EXAMINATION
Encouragement of regular BSE for self-detection of breast cancer symptoms, followed by breast specialist consultation:
- TEACHING BSE IN ISOLATION, results in *SPORADIC BSE,* which results in *SPORADIC SELF-DETECTION* of breast cancer symptoms, which results in *SPORADIC BREAST CANCER DETECTION* at physician's consultations
  (causes a false feeling of security)
- BSE BUILT INTO A COMPREHENSIVE SYSTEMATIC PROGRAMME, which includes personal instruction, a check on the regularity of BSE and an immediate breast specialist referral, results in *SYSTEMATIC BSE,* early *SELF-DETECTION OF SYMPTOMS* and *EARLY BREAST CANCER DETECTION* at a breast specialist's consultation
  (causes a feeling of security)

The aims of the programme

In response to the challenges presented at the end of the previous chapter and in order to meet different needs for a systematic search for breast cancer – both from the individual woman's point of view and from the public health agencie's point of view – I have designed a multidimensional BSE-centered programme for early detection of breast cancer. The aims of this programme are as follows:
- To reduce fears and pessimism associated with breast cancer
- To motivate women to take part in the multidimensional programme and to persist in performing BSE throughout their lives in a systematic and continuous manner
- To teach cautious BSE technique
- To teach what is normal for the individual women's breasts, and, consequently, to identify changes in the breasts, if such occur
- To arrange a direct link between a woman who detects breast cancer symptoms herself, and a breast specialist
- To reduce patient's delay and doctor's delay

- To ease the pressure on physicians in general, as well as breast specialists
- To implement the multidimensional programme in existing public health systems
- To reduce detection and treatment costs
- To enrol the medical decision making authorities and agencies in a programme which will ensure adequate health education, administration facilities, as well as breast specialists and equipment for competent medical diagnosis of breast cancer.

Health education aspects

A programme that would serve the aims indicated has to provide a system of action whereby the following requirements are fulfilled:
- Observable symptoms of the disease have to be noticed at an early stage
- The detection of symptoms should be followed up by further diagnostic procedures as soon as possible (e.g. mammography, ultrasound, etc.)
- An affirmative diagnosis should be followed by immediate treatment.

In order to fulfill the above requirements two categories of achievements are needed:
- Factors that can positively promote the fulfillment of the requirements (e.g. we should motivate women to perform BSE systematically and to notice observable signs of breast cancer)
- Factors that can eliminate frequently prevailing obstacles (e.g. we should reduce such fears and change negative attitudes which the individual woman might have).

The above overview, clearly demonstrates, that there is a need for a programme that is multidimensional enough to bring about a co-ordinated entity of action, within which all these different needs can be met.

Therefore, the programme that will now be described has been constructed as a multidimensional one, that would be able to meet the above requirements. Although it includes a few features of administratively technical nature, the major characteristics of the programme are genuinely educational.

The programme should be described as an entity, consisting of three major components:

a) Person-to-person interface (communication)
b) A feed-back system
c) A specialist referral system

Person-to-person communication

A medically trained key-person informs women in groups or individually about: background problems in breast cancer and detection of the disease, the structure of the actual information programme, the cautious BSE-technique and the name of the breast specialist who is selected for women reporting with symptoms. The main emphasis is on reassurance, on encouraging and motivating the women to follow the programme and prompt reporting of symptoms if such occur.

Basically, the medical informants involved in the information part of the programme should handle the related tasks as a part of their daily routine. They are to be recruited all over the country having their main tasks in different public health and other health related functions.

The feed-back system

In order to keep check on women's health behaviour regarding regular BSE, specially designed material is used. Each woman receives a calendar on which to record a whole year's monthly BSE examination dates. The calendar also has space in which details on how to contact the breast specialist, if symptoms occur. And it contains a summary description of the cautious BSE technique. The calendar serves as a tool in the communication between the key-person and a woman. At the end of each year it is to be handed back to the key-person.

The woman will then receive a new calendar for the following year, together with further information, both mass communication and person-to-person communication nature.

Development of the feedback system was influenced by several considerations. A yearly question and answer interview with a woman cannot immediately give reliable information as to her BSE behaviour. Her memory of what she did is likely to be vague. A written record is therefore essential. Indeed, her posession of the calendar will increase the likelihood of her motivation to perform regular BSE in the first place. The psychological benefits are of course obvious. When an interest is shown in notes made in their calendars, people feel that they are being carefully looked after and that they are not alone with their BSE. (I was strengthened in this conviction through my experience of an analogous person-to-person motivation and feed-back system for smoking cessation purposes). And lastly, the calendars cost very little to produce, yet offer a quick and easy way of getting behavioural information. There is thus no obstacle to their adoption within existing health services, where they can be handled by nurses. Moreover, the key-persons, by keeping a close annual check on individuals, are able to tailor the information in a more personal way for special needs or circumstances.

The specialist referral system

Breast specialists (experienced surgeons, radiologists, cytologists and oncologists) are selected to be in charge of women who detect symptoms themselves. They are to give diagnosis or make further referrals for diagnosis and treatment if necessary. As already mentioned, each woman's calendar has a note of the breast specialist with responsibility for her. This too is calculated to increase her sense of security, which will eliminate or at least reduce such anxiety that might make her hesitant when it comes to showing her symptoms to a physician. This psychological factor contributes substantially to minimizing patient's delay. The referral system further reduces patient's delay by eliminating the risk that the woman begins by contacting the wrong physician. This does, at the same time, eliminate such a doctor's delay that would occur as a result from the instruction of an extra, unnecessary step of referral from one physician to the next one. Basically, the breast specialists involved in the referral system should handle the related tasks as part of their daily routine. They are to be recruited all over a country.

Chapter III

The multidimensional programme in operation – a test project

General questions

Questions raised in testing the programme were:
- What did the women know, feel and do about breast cancer and early detection before joining the programme?
- Can knowledge be improved and a change in attitudes (fears) and behaviour (BSE) be brought about, such that women will be ready to take part in a long-term programme?
- Does age, formal education or occupation correlate with any such change?
- What are women's opinions about the programme?
- To what extent do women identify symptoms of breast cancer?
- How much can patient's delay and doctor's delay probably be reduced?
- Can more cases be detected with than without this kind of intervention?
- Can the mortality rate be reduced?
- What resources of facilities personnel, equipment and money would be needed for the permanent institutionalization of the programme?
- Could the programme be implemented in public health systems of other countries?
- How could the programme fit in with other types of detection programmes?

Material in the project

History of the project

From 1955 to 1968 the present author worked as a radiologist in the field of cancer detection and treatment, and from 1962 to 1973 as Chief Education Officer for the Cancer Society of Finland. Based on my previous work which included planning for early detection of cancer diseases it soon became clear to me that mass communication alone could not be relied on to motivate women to regular breast self-examination. tion.

In 1972 two nationwide Finnish women's organizations, Marttaliitto and Finlands Svenska Marthaförbund with altogether about 100000 members, were planning to have a "health project year", and consulted me to develop a programme, which, if successful, could be applied to the entire population. The field chosen was breast cancer and its early detection. The method developed was called the Mama Method, "Mama"being derived from both women's organization's names.

The project was planned to resemble health-care arrangements already institutionalized. The leaders of the organizations were aware that the programme was being tested for subsequent implementation in the public health service.

In 1974 the two organizations Marttaliitto (Finnish speaking) and Finlands Svenska Marthaförbund (Swedish speaking) founded co-operatively the "Martha 75th Year Jubilee Fund". A large contribution to the fund was made by The Social Insurance Institution of Finland, which enabled the necessary field work to be realized. The material which was used in the project by a key-person and myself and by the women enrolled in the programme was planned and prepared by me and paid partly by private donations to me and by grants to the Jubilee Fund. X-ray films for mammography examination of women who were expected to show up with self detected breast cancer symptoms, were paid for by private donation to me.

Running the Mama Project

In 1973 the test project got under way, first in one regional division of the organizations and then in others, with a two year's project in every region. At the outset myself and 19 other physicians (radiologists and surgeons) were asked to take part by arranging for consultations with symptomatic women and all the physicians accepted the invitation.

Particular regional divisions were selected where I acted as key-person and in one of them as the breast specialist selected in advance.

One nurse was personally trained by myself and was then employed by the women's organizations, acting as a key-person in the person-to-person interface phase as did myself.

The field work came to an end in 1974, apart from one area with 10000 women (the regional division of Turku) where it continued into 1975. The evaluation stage ended in 1980, when the five-year mortality figures became available and the present book was written (Gästrin 1973–1980).

The test group and the control group

Marttaliitto and Finlands Svenska Marthaförbund were founded over 80 years ago and have a very consistant membership of young, middle-aged and old women. Their regional and local leaders have a clear idea of who actually belongs to their divisions as active members (lists of members). Regional divisions have from about 1 000 to 10 000 members and they are divided into local chapters of about 50 to 100 members each.

The test group participants in the project consisted of 56 177 women, aged 20 to 80 years. They were members of the two women's organizations mentioned, constituting entire local chapters, not selected sample groups. The local chapters had an even geographical spread all over the country. The project participants thus represent a fair cross-section of the organization members. These women demonstrate such characteristics with respect to health, socio-economic status, formal education and occupation, that they seem to be fairly close to average conditions for the total of the female population.

At the initial planning of the project as project leader, I intended to adopt the traditional experiment/control group design, but the choice of a control group representing the general population was problematic.

Women outside the test group were likely to be influenced by the project's mass media information, so that there would not be any properly "non-exposed" group available.

I therefore decided to let the control group for the evaluation of clinical findings consist of the entire female population of Finland in 1972, which is the year before the project started. In 1972 the general population was still unaffected by the project's informative efforts. A subgroup consisting of one regional division, the rural area of Northern Carelia with 2 900 project participants, was chosen for careful supervision and control of certain test results.

When the project started the leaders of the local chapters of the women's organizations summoned their members to meetings, at which the key-person presented information as described earlier. Those members who had been unable to attend the meeting, were reached by follow-up contacts by the local leaders. They then kept a record of participants.

Each participant received a calendar for two year's use as well as the name and address of the breast specialist who was selected in advance and thus was in charge of every woman who detects symptoms of breast cancer herself.

Key-persons

The project leader and one nurse acted as key-persons. The nurse, who was employed full-time in the project, learned the contents of the information and the way of conveying information by first attending some information meetings conducted by myself as the project leader. I then prepared a teaching kit for the nurse, containing motivating and activating information for the women in the project, plus details of the feedback and referral systems. The information content passed on by myself as the project leader, and the nurse, was designed to be identical.

Volunteers

When the project started in each area, the leaders of the organizations arranged information meetings. They kept files on the women participating, and saw to the distribution of calendars. They also contacted local chapter members absent from the information meetings. They reminded participants now and then about the on-going programme.

Breast specialists

On the initiative of the project leader, myself and 19 other specialists in breast cancer (radiologists and surgeons), worked on a voluntary basis and in close co-operation with me in different parts of the country. No one of them worked full-time on the project: the consultations with symptomatic women were in addition to their normal routine. There was obviously no way of knowing in advance exactly how many women any one specialist might have to see, but they each knew the size of the regional divisions membership for which they assumed responsibility. They kept special files on project participants who showed up with symptoms, noting details of age, symptom, further examination, clinical diagnosis, PAD and treatment. These records were forwarded to the project leader at the end of the project.

In one part of Finland a screening programme was in operation for one year at the same time as this project (Soini 1977). But the physician

conducting that screening was also involved as one of the breast specialists in this project. Together with the author/project leader she made sure
that no newly detected case was registered twice.

Printed and other material

The teaching kit which was used by the key-person was planned and
written by me and the illustrations used for demonstration were drawn by
myself. Through conversations with several hundred women it became
clear that drawn illustrations were accepted better than photographs; the
main reason for this was that women could not personally identify with
photographs of other women. Therefore the project proceeded with
illustrations, which were later on redrawn by the artist Henrik Tikkanen.

The teaching kit used by the key-person comprised:
- A booklet containing the message: a lecture on breast cancer problems
  and solutions; comments on the misunderstandings and fears which
  prevent women from taking proper care of themselves; an outline of
  the need for a new solution on a global scale; a description of the
  multidimensional programme; a description for the use of hand-out
  material (calendars); a description of cautious BSE technique; and
  what to do if symptoms of breast cancer occur
- Slides to go with the lecture
- A poster designed to act as a demonstration and reminder
  The materials used by every woman in the project were:
- A copy of the calendar
- Questionnaires concerning personal background factors
- Polls regarding their opinions of the project

During the project these three different items used by the project
participants were put together on one piece of paper, which was to be
returned after the end of the project. The calendar consists of:
- A real calendar for monthly notes about BSE date
- Space for writing down the name of the breast specialist
- A repetition of the cautious BSE technique

Mass media

The mass media took part, sometimes on the invitation of the project
leader, sometimes on their own initiative. When the project was started
in each region, interviews for the radio, TV and the press were made with

the key-persons and members of the women's organiations. This type of communication then occured often, in all regions.

Furthermore, a special television spot was designed by the project leader to motivate and remind members of the women's organizations to go on with the project. This spot was shown 30 times all over the country on the national TV-network. This was particularly important in areas with long distances between members and their leaders.

Collection and analysis of data

Psychological effects

In addition to the main components of the programme, the test project also had certain extra features designed to measure something of its psychological effect: interviews before and after entering this programme; and questionnaires and opinion polls which were distributed to all participants together with the calendars at the initial information meeting and returned to the project leader two years later.

The interviews were carried out with a subgroup including 2 900 participants from Northern Carelia. The majority of these women took part in the interviews. 74 % of them returned their questionnaires and calendars. In the following sections on Knowledge, Attitudes, Opinions and Behaviour before and after entering this programme the findings are derived from analysis of the interviews and of the printed material returned by those belonging to the interview group.

Knowledge

Before the initial information meeting the 2 900 women from Northern Carelia (1974) were asked in groups of 30 to 50 women each, whether they prior to this project had known about the necessity of regular BSE. An interview like this had not previously been made in Finland; in the areas concerned women had for about 40 years received brochures regarding breast cancer, made by the Finnish Cancer Society and distributed in different ways as e.g. in connection with Pap-tests (these brochures are similar to those of e.g. The American Cancer Society).

The answers "yes" or "no" were recorded and expressed in percentages of the women interviewed.

About 100 % of the women interviewed answered that they did know about the necessity of regular monthly BSE. This indicates that previously prevailing mass communication for health education about BSE had influenced knowledge.

Attitudes and opinions before and after entering the Mama Programme

Before the information meeting the respondents were asked in groups of 30 to 50 women about their attitudes and opinions regarding present health education, different kinds of information and communication, fears, beliefs, BSE and breast cancer. What was shown was very much like the author's experiences in connection with previous health education for BSE. As for the attitudes of women themselves, they have already accepted breast cancer information for several decades, and the present author's experience suggests that they are very motivated for the type of programme proposed here. Asked if they would prefer to live a shorter time with breast cancer or a longer time with it diagnosed and treated, nearly every woman opts for the latter. Some women said that they would never let a breast be removed but they added that this was their opinion in a situation when they did not have to choose. Women earlier treated said that their attitudes changed in this matter within a few minutes of their doctors telling them that they needed an operation for breast cancer. They chose to live in hope of a longer life, even if the quality of life had to change in some respects. Very few women in the vulnerable age group were so concerned about their breasts that they wanted to keep them at any price. Women have a complex web of desires and fears of which breast cancer is only a part, and the treatment of breast cancer definitely solves more problems than it creates. Women know, too, that surgery nowadays can be less incapacitating than it used to be. So they are keen to achieve the early diagnosis that is the precondition for this.

The interviews indicated that only a very small fraction of the women seemed to suffer from anxieties. Most of them said that uncertainty makes them passive, so that BSE had not become a regular habit. Most of them did know about the cautious BSE technique and what to look for but they did not know which physician to contact with breast cancer symptoms. They thought that the gynaecologist was the expert physician in breast cancer. They also thought that their breasts were frequently enough examined by nurses in connection with screenings for cervical cancer. The interviews also indicated that the women were very responsive to the message given in the programme. They were apparently motivated to adopt something new in the early detection of breast cancer.

Immediately after the initial information the same 2 900 project participants were asked if the information at the meeting had made for anxieties or for greater sense of security. All women who explained their feelings said that they felt more secure.

According to plans, the participants received initial person-to-person information from a key-person; they had been exposed to the TV spot reminding them to keep on with the programme; and they had also been reminded by a volunteer from the organization. As will be seen, most of them responded to this battery of communication by adopting regular BSE behaviour 12 times in a row during a year.

The first question asked was which component of the information that had been given had the most effect on motivation to proceed with the programme. Of those who were reached by all three types of information, 43 % thought that person-to-person interface was most effective, 22 % the TV reminder, and 9 % the volunteer reminder. Of those who had not attended the key-person's information meeting, 35 % thought that the TV spot was most important, and 15 % the volunteer reminder.

There is thus little doubt that the person-to-person information worked best, and that television can also be a useful tool when the speaker is seen to be a reliable informant. The same thing was shown by the Danish and Australian television campaigns mentioned in Chapter I. As also noted, however, the effect of a television spot is limited to the period during which it is actually transmitted.

The second question asked was whether the calendar itself had been particularly important as a stimulus to regular BSE. The significance of the calendar for feed-back purposes had been thoroughly explained at the information meeting, and the question was deliberately phrased as a "leading question" so as to make the women think about its role still further. Of the project participants who had attended the information meeting, 81 % thought the calendar was very important. Of those who had not attended the information meeting, and who had consequently not heard its role fully explained, 67 % thought it was very important. Factors of formal education, occupation and age did not seem to influence these answers.

Lastly, from conversations with many individual women in the project it became clear that one feature of the programme which greatly enhanced the motivation to proceed with the programme was the direct link with a named breast specialist. The women knew that if they did find a symptom they would immediately receive expert personalized attention.

Behaviour before and after entering the Mama Programme

Out of 2 900 project participants interviewed before the start of the project, about 100 % knew that BSE should be performed every month, according to the interviews described but only 0–2 % of them claimed that they themselves practised it regularly. In other words, previously used methods of information (mostly mass communication) had conveyed the message and influenced knowledge without influencing behaviour.

At the end of the project, the author/project leader received the calendars back and was thus able to make an assessment of behavioural changes during the programme. Of those who had received information and calendars, 68 % had examined their breasts themselves for 12 months in a row during the first project year. Out of those, who had received person-to-person interface by a medical informant at the initial information meeting, 87 % of those who had returned their calendars had examined their breasts for 12 months in a row.

The figures regarding behaviour before and after entering the Mama Programme are extremely rough with respect to formal precision. The comparison is therefore equally unprecise in terms of figure values. However, when the raw figures to be compared are in order of 1 respectively 68 %, we do not need too stringent formal precision to find the difference valid as an expression of a significant change.

The women's acceptance of the programme clearly coincided with a behavioural change, which can most probably be accounted for by the personalized information by a medical informant.

A further study was made of the relation between the change in BSE behaviour and formal education, occupation and age. The findings were as follows:

		Percentage of women who performed BSE 12 times in a row
Formal education	primary school	75
	secondary school	79
	college or university	86
Occupation	housewife	77
	employed	77
Age	≤29	73
	30–44	80
	45–59	76
	60–74	67
	≥75	38

This seems to suggest that neither a woman's level of education nor her status as housewife or employee had much to do with her response to the message. Women 30 to 44 years of age had been most active in performing BSE 12 times in a row. With advancing age, and especially among women over 75, less BSE activity took place.

Some long-term data

The author/project leader was interested to know whether the sense of security remained more or less constant throughout the project period and after the project had ended. Individual interviews were therefore conducted with 100 project participants at the author's breast specialist office, to which 230 symptomatic women had reported, 19 of them being newly diagnosed breast cancer patients within the first project year. Nearly all of them stated that the multidimensional programme had promoted a sustained sense of security.

Five years after the project had ended letters were sent out to all new breast cancer patients detected within this project's first year in the whole country. The project leader received answers from 55 % indicating that all of them felt a sense of security.

Opinions of the key-persons and the breast specialists

The impression of both key-persons and breast specialists are also of some interest, since one of the project's aims was to test the new programme for implementation in existing public health care systems with existing personnel.

The key-persons thought the informative programme offered a valuable way of approaching the large female population. They noticed that it seemed to reassure women. And they were very well received, which encouraged and motivated them in their work.

The attitudes of the breast specialists in the programme were equally positive. They felt the referral system worked well, and noted that the workload on them was small and that the detection rate for this group was high. They therefore thought the multidimensional programme had considerable potential as a model for detection, and would themselves have liked to reach more women in this simple way.

Clinical effects

To indicate whether the Mama Programme brought about earlier diagnosis, details will soon be given of actual rate of diagnosis, compared to the expected rate, the age of the patients, the proportion of cases with and without axillary spread and the 5-year mortality rate. All these variables can provide criteria of "true" early diagnosis.

Definitions

Those cases of breast cancer which are here described as cases first discovered in the project satisfy the following criteria: A project participant has, as a result of this programme, carried out BSE, detected some of the symptoms mentioned, shown them to the project breast specialist, and has been diagnosed as a new breast cancer case.

All cases which came to the attention of the project leader through the project's breast specialists have been confirmed as newly discovered cases by checking with the hospital where the patient was treated and with the files of The Finnish Cancer Registry.

The participants who within 12 months of the initial information meeting showed up with self-detected symptoms and were diagnosed as breast cancer cases are here called patients of the first project year. The participants who showed up and received a diagnosis during the second twelve-month period are here called patients of the second project year.

In what follows only two different stages of the tumour are distinguished: cases with negative axillary lymph nodes (local cases) and cases with positive axillary lymph nodes.

For every newly detected case the project leader has checked date of clinical diagnosis, the stage of the tumour, and the histopathologic diagnosis with the records of the hospitals where the patients were treated and with the files of The Finnish Cancer Registry.

The project leader obtained details about the five year mortality of the project's newly diagnosed cases during the first project year by sending each patient a personal letter five years after she received her clinical diagnosis. Replies have been received from the patients themselves or their next of kin. The project leader has checked all details with the official registers of population.

Five year mortality for the patients who received their diagnosis during the second project year has not been assessed.

Patient's delay

In the present project, it was nearly always possible to specify the time at which a project participant received information from the key-person, the time at which she detected a symptom herself, and the time at which she consulted a breast specialist in the project. These details derive from the calendars, from the specialists' files, and from the records of The Finnish Cancer Registry, and they are as follows:

Percentage of women who reported symptoms which later were shown to be breast cancer

within 0–30 days	within 2–3 Mo.	within 4–5 Mo.	within 6–7 Mo.	within 8–9 Mo.	within 10–11 Mo.	within 12 Mo.	un-known
44.3	18.5	6.2	7.2	1.0	3.1	6.2	13.5

The project thus seems to have motivated women to delay very little. 63 % reported their symptoms within three months and 44.3 % within a month. The results indicate that patient's delay was smaller than in earlier studies. Most of the women were motivated to contact the breast specialist after only short delay.

The project leader worked herself as one of the breast specialists in the project handling participants from the Uusimaa region.

Having established cooperation with another radiologist and a surgeon, arrangements for consultations were made at the out patient clinic of The Cancer Society of Finland. The group for whom this team of breast specialists had responsibility consisted of 10 000 women, who received information and the calendars in January 1973. Two hundred and thirty project participants appeared within 12 months with symptoms detected by regular BSE starting in January 1973. All of these showed up within one month after self-detection of symptoms.

Doctor's delay

There was practically no doctor's delay within the project. The specialists took women into their care within one week after appointment. The only slight exceptions were caused by summer holidays and by the emigration of one specialist while the project was still in operation.

Patient's show-up

Of the 56 177 women participating in the total project, within twelve months after the initial information meeting 750 (i.e. 1.3 %) reported with symptoms to a breast specialist. Roughly 40 women reported on average to each of the 20 breast specialists. Of those women who consulted a breast specialist during the first project year about every eighth was actually a new breast cancer case. Out of the 750 women who showed up and were not diagnosed as new breast cancer cases, a few were checked at further visits, and some of them were diagnosed as cases during the project's second year. During the second year of the project about 300 project participants reported with symptoms. Roughly 0.5 % of them consulted a breast specialist during that year, and of these about every ninth was actually a new breast cancer case. The physicians also noted over 30 recurrences, but these are not taken up in the figures which follow.

The work load on the physicians was small in view of the number of new cases detected.

The women who showed up with symptoms and then proved to be newly detected breast cancer cases had found one of the typical symptoms that can be detected by self-examination, e.g. retraction of the skin or the nipple (about 45 %), lumps of different size (about 45 %) and about 10 % being other symptoms that can be detected by women themselves.

In the group handled by the author there were 19 new cases, two of which had only retraction of the skin. The intraductal carcinomas found by self-palpation were smaller than 1 cm in diameter.

Diagnostic data

The expected incidence of breast cancer for the entire project group was calculated by applying age-specific rates for the national population in 1972, as derived from publications of The Finnish Cancer Registry (Cancer Incidence in Finland 1972, Helsinki 1975) to the number of project women estimated to be in each age group. This estimate has been based on the assumption that the age distribution of the total project group is similar to that of the total group of organization members so as revealed by a survey made of the women's organizations in 1975. This assumption seems reasonable because the local chapters participated in the project in their entirety and because participating local chapters had an even distribution geographically. But the lack of exact age data does of course limit the precision of the calculations.

According to the above calculations the expected number of new breast cancer cases would have been 51.3 in one year for the group of total 56 177 women. The actual number of cases diagnosed in that group during the first year of the project was 90. During the second year of the project 35 new cases were detected. This indicates that during the first project year a number of new breast cancer cases had obviously been detected which would not have been detected until later without this intervention.

It should be noted that this pattern of development over a period of time fits well into the picture that serves as the traditionally accepted criterion for the successfulness of a screening programme for early detection: during the first year a rise above initial level; during the next year a drop below initial level.

Another observation could be done with regard to the group handled by the author herself. The monthly distribution after the initial information meeting was a follows:

Number of new breast cancer cases each month	Jan	Feb	Mar	Apr	May	June	Jul	Aug	Sept	Oct	Nov	Dec
	6	0	2	4	2	1	0	0	2	0	1	1

Thus more than two thirds of the new cases were detected within the first six months. This uneven distribution of diagnosis over the year supports the hypothesis that there were a good deal previously "hidden" cases that were detected right at the start of the programme.

The programme's capacity to pick up hidden cases is illustrated from another angle in the data from the Northern Carelian subgroup. This region offered the following picture:

Northern Carelia is an area, where the borders of the regional division of the organization correspond with those of governmental administration and figures made up by The Finnish Cancer Registry. The age distribution of the participants is rather equivalent to that of the normal female population in that region.

In the year before the project in this low-incidence area the rate of diagnosis was 0.64 cases per 1 000 women. In the first project year 79 of the area's 2 900 participants showed up with self-detected symptoms and 9 proved to be new cases. This corresponds to a rate of diagnosis of 3.1 per 1 000 women.

The very high ratio between observed and expected rate of diagnosis from the very region where the programme activities could be best performed gives a rather favourable indication of the efficiency of the programme.

The ratio between observed and expected rate of diagnosis deserves being specifically studied with respect to age. For the first project year the figures were as follows in the total project group:

The ratio between observed and expected cases; first year

Age	20–34	35–44	45–54	55–64	≥65	Total
Number of cases expected per year	0.3	4.2	11.3	17.1	18.4	51.3
Number of observed cases in first project year		12	25	27	26	90
"Incidence ratio" (observed/expected)	0	2.9	2.2	1.6	1.4	1.8

The rate of diagnosis was higher than expected in every single age group. (It should be noted that the "incidence ratio" for the total group given here is not a simple average of the values in each age-group, since the age-groups are made up of different numbers of individuals). This consistency of pattern supports the suggestion that the intervention by the programme has been the major factor behind the difference. Further, the "incidence ratio" (observed/expected) was especially high in the age group 35 to 44 years and then decreased with increasing age. This reflects the fact that the cases diagnosed in the project have a lower median age (56 years) than those (about 61 years) in the general population (age-adjusted to the project group). This difference in median age again suggests that cases detected in the project represent an earlier average stage of detection than the one in the uninfluenced, general population.

Of the 90 new cases in the entire project's first year there were 63 cases with negative axillary lymph nodes (70 %), and 27 cases with positive axillary lymph nodes (30 %). In 4 cases there was an intraductal carcinoma; the expected figure was about 2. The number of cases with axillary lymph nodes was significantly lower than expected.

Age	35–44	45–54	55–64	65–74	≥75	Total
Cases in 1st project year	12	25	27	20	6	90
Negative axillary lymph nodes	8	17	19	15	4	63
Positive axillary lymph nodes	4	8	8	5	2	27

According to unpublished data from The Finnish Cancer Registry 52 % of all new Finnish cases of breast cancer in 1973 had positive axillary lymph nodes. This would give a figure of 27 expected axillary spreads for the project group, which was precisely the number actually found. Thus it is at least conceivable that all the "extra" cases established within the project were "local cases", i.e. cases with negative axillary lymph nodes.

This observation does again provide evidence suggesting that the programme activities do result in an early detection.

Mortality

All the detected cases were treated with mastectomy, and some with radiotherapy as well, but an account of this is not included here. However, a comparison of the mortality rate in the project group with the rate otherwise to be expected is accounted in the following.

Mortality data for breast cancer in Finland has been published by The Finnish Cancer Registry for many years. During the period 1966 to 1970 the mortality rate five years after diagnosis for all breast cancer patients was on an average 45 % (Teppo et al. 1975). In the project, the rate was 31 %. Out of the 90 new cases in the project's first year 28 patients died within five years.

A break-down in age groups is given in the table below:

Deaths within 5 years after diagnosis (all cases)

Age at diagnosis	35–44	45–54	55–64	≥65	Total
Number of breast cancers	12	25	27	26	90
Cause of death known to be breast cancer	1	5	4	5	15
Cause of death unknown	–	6	2	5	13

The Finnish Cancer Registry has according to figures from Finland 1956–1970 calculated an expected five-year mortality rate for the cases with negative axillary lymph nodes in this project for the various age-groups (Hakulinen 1980). A comparison with the mortality rates actually occuring is as follows:

Deaths within 5 years after diagnosis (local cases)

Age	35–44	45–54	55–64	≥65	Total
Expected deaths in 5 years	2.15	5.75	8.35	12.48	28
Observed deaths within 5 years after diagnosis	0	6	3	6	15

Even the project group's local cases demonstrate significantly lower mortality than expected. This suggests that these cases represent a still less advanced stage of tumour development than the average one among the local cases in an intervention free population.

Five-year mortality figures cannot be stated as entirely sufficient indication that this project was really able to postpone death. When the twenty-year figures become available the picture will be much clearer.

Nevertheless, the five-year figures do begin to have a certain weight when taken into conjunction with three of the project's other findings: the high proportion of cases with negative axillary lymph nodes; the low median age of the detected new cases; and the higher than usual proportion of intraductal cases. It could finally be noted that, when speaking of measures of a programme's effect, the best single one so far available would most probably be the proportion of the detected cases that have negative axillary lymph nodes.

Costs

Although no special cost-benefit analysis has been carried out, a few observations should nevertheless be of interest. As already noted, during the first year only 750 of the 56 177 participants reported to the 20 specialists, and 90 of this 750 proved to be new breast cancer cases; in other words, every specialist was consulted by roughly 40 women, of whom roughly one in ten was a new case for an entire group of 56 177 women covered.

The essential costs were in communication. Information meetings had to be arranged, the participants had to travel to meetings, the nurse had a salary, and the calendar and other materials had to be produced. Since the programme was intended for subsequent implementation into a public health system, estimates were made of what this would cost. If information meetings were organized as part of normal public health care activities and in places of employment they would cost very little. Within the public health system and at many places of employment, there are already salaried staff who could work as key-persons. If women attend the meetings while at their place of work they would have no travel costs. And the costs for the calendar etc. are in any case negligible.

At a time when none of the potential advantages of the public health system could yet be drawn on, the information costs for each woman informed in the project was $ 0.50, and for each newly diagnosed case $ 200. This second figure is about a tenth or a twentieth of the costs involved for each new case as compared with today's screening programmes.

Fringe effects in Finland

The project described in this chapter has entailed a number of activities giving rise to "fringe effects" in Finland from 1973 and onwards. This section will describe such activities and discuss what effects they and other projects might have had on the registered rate of diagnosis of breast cancer in Finland after 1972.

Activities entailed by the project

In 1973 when the project started in the regions Uusimaa and Häme where 10000 women were enrolled, there was a great interest aroused by mass media such as TV, women's magazines, etc. Interest was also aroused in women who were relatives to or friends of the project participants being about another 10000. These women contacted project participants, women's organization leaders or the project leader (who was the key-person and the breast specialist of that very region), some women contacted "own physicians". Around 30 new breast cancer cases in women who were outside the project group came to the project-leader's attention. No one of these cases are published by the present author as attributed to the Mama Project, but they will be included in the official cancer statistics for the year 1973.

In 1974, when the project was running in Northern Carelia, there were relatives and friends of the project group, women who wanted to join a similar programme as did the project group women. These women outside the project group were told by the project participants, by the leader's of the women's organizations and by the key-person (the projec-leader) that they could contact the breast specialist in the programme. The breast specialist of that very area reported 7 new cases in the project group as already reported in this book, but there were 9 cases in relatives and friends who did show up because of their knowledge about and interest in this programme. These 9 cases are not published by the present author as attributed to her Mama Project, but they will be included in the official cancer statistics for the year 1974.

In 1974 an invitation was issued through the mass media to the total of 6000 women over 35 years of age on the Åland Islands (which constitute one of the geographical regions of Finland but form an administratively independent, home-ruled province). Their voluntary participation was urged in a project of the same kind as the original Mama Project. The initiative was taken care of by a local health organization, Folkhälsan på Åland. The author arranged a referral link with a breast specialist and the organization employed a part-time nurse/key-person to give person-to-person information in groups and to individuals. The television spot about breast cancer being shown in the Finnish mainland could not be seen in Åland, so that this is an interesting case of what can be done without television. The radio and press, on the other hand, gave the fullest coverage. Of the 6000 women invited, 3900 participated. Since this group was self-selected the results are not a valid measure of the programme's potential for Åland. Of the 3900 calendars distributed, 21 % were returned. Before the programme started, interviews showed that 0–2 % of the women had previously carried out BSE regularly. The calendars returned showed that 18 % of the programme participants adopted monthly BSE 12 times in a row during one year. As in the main test project, we see that quite a substantial behavioural change occured.

In 1972 there were 3 new cases of breast cancer in Åland, and in 1973, 6 new cases. In 1974, which was the year of the Åland project, 7 cases were newly detected within the 3900 project women alone. As in the main test project, this was roughly twice the expectation for the group. As in the main project, too, the programme seemed to reveal the disease in younger women than usual.

According to official statistics of The Finnish Cancer Registry, in Åland as a whole there were 9 new cases in 1974 (including the project's 7). Form the year after the Åland project, the number of cases diagnosed in Åland fell to 5, which again corresponds to the pattern in the main project. All the cases in the Åland project were local cases without positive axillary lymph nodes. One was an intraductal carcinoma. No one of these cases are published by the present author as attributed to the Mama Project, but they will be included in the official cancer statistics for the year 1974.

In 1974 on the initiative of the present author a television spot was prepared reminding women participating in the Mama Project. It lasted 1 1/2 minutes and was shown on the national TV-network 30 times during 1974. Thereby the message of the TV-spot reached also women outside the project group. The side effects to the main project being seen as a result of this TV-project was as follows: The author/project-leader received about 50–70 telephone calls from women all over the country not belonging to the project, who told how, as a result of the TV-programme, they had examined themselves just once and immediately found symptoms that were at a following medical examination diagnosed to be breast cancer. No one of these cases are published by the present author as attributed to the Mama Project, but they will be included in the official cancer statistics for the year 1974.

Non project related activities

Just as the above mentioned activities entailed by the project can have influenced the rate of detection of breast cancer in Finland since 1973, there are even other activities that might also have done so:

- Information and counseling that was distributed as usual by The Finnish Cancer Society in a multitude of ways since 40 years (the present author/project leader of the Mama Project was Chief of Education of the Cancer Society 1962–1973). After the Mama Project results were published by the author in Finland and other countries, societies have publically supported the importance of person-to-person communication.
- Screening programme of the City of Tampere in Finland involving 20 644 women; about 30 new breast cancer cases were detected in this project, which was conducted by Dr. Irma Soini in co-operation with the Cancer Association of Tampere and which has been evaluated (Soini 1977).

Breast cancer statistics in Finland

Predictions were made by The Finnish Cancer Registry in 1973 for the breast cancer incidence in 1980. The prediction suggested that the incidence in Finland would rise, as in most countries, but not very steeply, between 1 100 and 1 400 new cases in 1980 (Teppo et al. 1973).

What actually happened was an increase from 1 126 new cases in 1972 to 1 406 new cases already in 1976. New predictions were made by The Finnish Cancer Registry in 1980, suggesting that the number of new registered breast cancer cases would rise to about 1 658 in 1985 (Holsti 1980).

New cases of breast cancer annually registered in Finland

(The Mama Project was tested 1973–1975 and the Mama Programme has been introduced step by step in the existing health care system since 1975)

Number of registred breast cancer cases in Finland	1972	1973	1974	1975	1976	1977	1978	1979	1980
	1 126	1 301	1 368	1 304	1 406	1 439			

Since the actual rate of diagnosis seems to exceed the predicted one, it would be reasonable to look for factors that can have influenced the rate of diagnosis although not being known beforehand and, consequently, not taken into account when the predictions were calculated. As a matter of fact the Mama Project, the fringe effects of the Mama Project, and the implementation of the Mama Programme into the existing health care system since 1975 may constitue such influences.

Further investigations would be needed to determine to what extent these effects can explain the excess rate of diagnosis, and some ideas will be given in connection with interviews performed by The Finnish National Board of Health concerning opinions among women in the Finnish female population and among breast cancer patients (p. 69).

Chapter IV

Implementation of the Mama Programme into public health systems

Initiatives for implementation

National level

In 1975 the Finnish women's organizations Marttaliitto and Finlands Svenska Marthaförbund made a request to the Finnish National Board of Health that the programme, now tested, should be offered to all women in all areas of the country. In 1975 the Finnish National Board of Health gave recommendations to all community health centers, that all women in connection with different medical check-ups should be motivated to perform regular BSE.

Since 1975 training courses on different levels and in nursing schools have taken place in order to motivate and prepare key-persons for their role in the Mama Programme; training has been prepared by the present author.

The material for key-persons (teaching kit) and for women enrolled in the Mama Programme (calendars) has been prepared by the present author.

Much is done in order to keep the programme going without interruptions, without deteriorating into short-term campaigns, and without losing its vital multidimensionality.

The annual participation in the programme rose from about 50000 in 1975 to more than 100000 in 1980, i.e. roughly one tenth of the adult Finnish female population. It is not known to what extent the same individuals persist respective to which extent old participants are replaced by new ones. The information and surveillance activities are handled by nurses and some physicans as part of their daily routine in public health functions (at maternity centers, post-natal check-ups, screenings for cervical cancer, etc.), in schools and universities, at places of work, in women's organizations, pensioners groups, gymnastic groups, etc. The breast specialists enrolled to take care of women who detect symptoms themselves are surgeons and radiologists dealing with these tasks at their usual offices in hospital clinics, out-patients clinics, University Clinics, private clinics, etc.

In 1977 the leaders of the women's organizations Marttaliitto and Finlands Svenska Marthaförbund, who had taken the initiative to request the implementation of the programme of the test-project, contacted all community health authorities in the whole of Finland and recommended to them that this programme should be offered to every woman disregarding living area or other circumstances.

In 1979 the National Board of Health in Finland recommended to all health centers that this programme should be offered to women in the whole country with the public health system serving as the channel for the information, follow-up and linkage to breast specialists (Recommendation 6191/02/79).

In 1979, Seppo Vihtonen, a programme chief of the Finnish State Television Company, asked the present author to prepare and to act in a new television spot for the national TV-network. Two different TV-spots were prepared; one of them directed towards decision-makers and key-persons, the other one towards women at large in the whole of the country.

Since the training of nurses, the recommendation of the Finnish National Board of Health and the TV spots began appearing in 1980, the author has again received telephone calles, just as in 1974 regarding new detected breast cancer cases on the basis of self-detection of symptoms in this programme. Some are from women who are enrolled in regular programmes and some from women who have detected symptoms of breast cancer as a result of the television spots.

In Finland and some parts of Sweden the Mama Programme has been permanently established. So far, those taking the initiative have turned for practical advice to the present author, who has produced a teaching-kit for the key-persons and the calendars for regular use and yearly exchange. Unable to evaluate all different practical examples of programmes in detail, the author has nevertheless kept an eye on the main lines of development, which give a clearer idea of the programme's wider potential for different countries and different systems. Some examples will perhaps help to suggest this.

County level

In 1974 the Finnish National Board of Health made Mikkeli County the object of an experimental study. The aim was to see how the programme might be implemented on county level. The author trained the key-persons in co-operation with the Chief Medical Officer of Mikkeli County, Dr. Tapani Lyyra. The initiatives in the various districts were dependent on the local decision makers, though they received written recommendations from the county central administration. The entire female population of the county by no means took part, but in those women that did, one out of every five who visited the physician with self-detected breast cancer symptoms within the programme was a new breast cancer case (Lyyra 1979).

If the provision of materials and training of key-persons are taken care of centrally and for an entire county, the programme on the district level will clearly be very inexpensive. Counties can thus make plans that will be geographically complete, and that will provide continuous coverage.

Major employer

In 1975, after the publication of the test-project's results, the author was approached by the authorities responsible for health care of employees of the City of Helsinki. With 15 600 women under their surveillance, they invited the author to train 25 nurses who would operate as key-persons with the help of the teaching-kit including a manual somewhat similar to parts of the present book. The calendars had the same format as in the test-project. The multidimensional programme worked well, conducted by motivated key-persons.

To some extent, women living in the nation's capital preferred to contact breast specialists "of their own" outside the scheme. Nevertheless, the number reporting to breast specialists within the scheme was in proportion with the results in the main test-project. So was the number of newly diagnosed breast cancer cases.

In connection with screening for cervical cancer

In the Turku region of Finland the test-project of the present author with about 10 000 women ended in 1975. During the present author's test-project in 1974–1975 interviews had been made among those 10 000 project participants about their present BSE habit. These interviews showed that only about 2 % performed BSE once a month and the percentage increased to about 50 during the course of the project.

In this same region the author, on the initiative of The Finnish National Board of Health, trained key-persons to carry out the programme in a fully systematic way and in different public health functions. In co-operation with decision-makers of the Turku region in 1975 the present author trained altogether about 500 key-persons and since then the region has ordered about 10 000 calendars per year for the implementation of the programme in different contexts within the Turku regions health system. Thus a large amount of women have already been involved within different schemes in the region from 1975 to 1980.

One scheme in particular within the Turku operations deserves a special note: the health counseling that takes place in connection with the screening for cervical cancer. In 1977 in connection with these screenings 10 037 women were taught BSE and received calendars designed by the present author. The women were urged to hand them back at yearly intervals to the communal health centers or to the out-patient clinic of the local cancer organization, where the cervical screening had taken place. In 1977 interviews were made with women participating in this screening scheme for cervical cancer. From this interview it became clear that 56 % of the women interviewed had performed BSE at least once a year and 50 % performed BSE between 6 and 12 times a year; a remarkable increase compared to 1974; this may reflect the influence of the test-project in 1974 to 1975, the repeated television spot and the work made in different schemes by about 500 trained key-persons in the Turku region, that has taken place since 1975, supported by the informative efforts that were made in connection to the screening programme.

The activities of the Turku scheme have been checked for the years 1977–1978 by the organizers of the screening for cervical cancer. During the first year of that scheme only 12.2 % of the women enrolled in the cervical screenings handed back their calendars as intended. By physical and mammography examination combined with the breast self-examination programme in that scheme, 1.7 new cases per 1 000 women were registered, which is more than expected (Räsänen et al. 1980).

As a comment on this result, one might stress that if the contact between the key-persons and the women in the scheme could be intense and continuous as the breast self-examination programme described is intended to be, this sort of channel could be one of the most effective of all the channels available in order to make women perform a self-control practice that is frequent enough.

In a women's gymnastic group

An initiative towards the programme was taken in 1977 by a gymnastic teacher who leads a housewive's gymnastic group at an institute for adult education. She obtained the teaching-kit with the manual and the calendars through the present author, and it was easy to arrange breast specialist consultations since the number likely to report per year was very low; the group consisted of 37 women. Of these, 36 returned their calendars for scrutiny after a year and then received new ones. As a result of the first year's programme, one woman found a breast cancer symptom herself, showed up immediately at the breast specialist's consultation, was treated, and then continued in the gymnastic group.

In this programme the key-person has been very active since 1977 and thus the little group took a special interest in the programme.

In a women's organization

A scheme within the Turku operations is a Mama Programme in a group of women belonging to the Martha organizations which began again with a programme in 1980, still continuing in 1981.

In a group of about 200 women, during one year 2 new breast cancer cases were detected starting with self-detection of symptoms and which were then confirmed as breast cancer cases at a breast specialist's consultation selected in advance (Serén 1981).

Interviews with women regarding BSE

Interviews regarding the acceptance of BSE on a regular basis 5 years after the implementation of the Mama Method have been made by health agencies and others.

In 1980 on the initiative of the Finnish National Board of Health a telephone-interview was made with about 1 000 women. The women were asked about BSE-related tasks. The answers were as follows:
– approx. 90 % thought BSE is important
– approx. 40 % claimed to perform BSE on a regular monthly basis
– approx. 31 % had learned the BSE-technique from the television spot prepared by the present author and 34 % by interface communication through a medically trained person (Elovainio 1980).

In 1980 an interview was made in Finland with 258 breast cancer patients regarding breast cancer related questions. The majority of the breast cancer patients had known about the necessity of BSE previous to their own illness and they claimed that the Mama Method was one of the main reasons for their performance of BSE on a regular basis (Mäntylä 1980). The findings in these interviews made after the implementation of the Mama Programme into public health care systems fit well together with the experiences of the present author.

The adoption of non-evaluated variants of the Mama Programme

When the results of the Finnish Mama Project became known, the present author was requested to plan a programme, to train key-persons and to prepare a manual for a region in a country outside Finland. There were more than half a million women in the actual province. At the last moment, however, some administrators altered the original intention, thus introducing a programme variant which was deprived of substancial components and that had not been previously evaluated. The calendar, the main instrument in person-to-person communication and the feed-back system was left out and key-persons were not taught about the reassuring information programme evaluated in the test-project. Instead, their training focused on: pedogogical methods; facts about breast cancer; psychological aspects; emotional reactions to breast cancer; the implications of losing a breast; psychological defense; psychological crisis; psychological obstacles to the teaching of BSE, etc.

A special obstacle was that undue emphasis was given to the view that breasts are "sexual organs" whose loss leaves a woman quite inconsolable. The key-persons trained were almost convinced that their task would make women anxious. Many of them were further negatively influenced by their own experiences of helplessness in nursing dying cancer patients; half of them never even examined their own breasts, for fear of what they might find. They thus had no firm ground from which to counter the target group's fears. And the women taught did not receive the necessary support and encouragement and they felt lonely with their BSE (Gyllensköld 1979).

Again, a variant of the programme tested was tried in another region. Material from the author's programme was studied in the region. A programme was used on the television in what was called "propaganda" for BSE. Certain calendars were distributed, but without any inbuilt feed-back system. Consultations were to be conducted at already existing "breast clinics".

The result of this programme variant was that women streamed to oncological consultations, in particular young women, and in such huge numbers that it was impossible to cope with them and the organizers tried to stop the programme (Hallberg 1979).

As already mentioned, in the multidimensional programme described in the present book the person-to-person communication safeguards this unnecessary pressure.

So, although some local refinements or adaptations of detail may be possible or even necessary, the central three elements of the multidimensional programme entity should be regarded as absolutely essential – the person-to-person communication, the feed-back system and the specialist referral system.

Operational viewpoints

Channels and initiatives

The programme's considerable benefits are entirely dependent on its multidimensional character being most carefully safeguarded. The three components, person-to-person communication through a key-person, surveillance and feed-back through the calendars, and specialist referral, have been tested, not separately, but as a coherent entity. So far the programme has interested decision makers and physicians in many countries in different parts of the world, not least because it seems to be adaptable to different systems, including different political systems. And it does not matter whether the key-persons are employed by state, district or some other body. They can fulfil their vital role – continuous personal information and feed-back – in any case.

The programme can be implemented on either a national, regional or local level. But in every case the first step must be to analyse the possible channels of communication in existing health systems and the availability of breast specialists.

The important point in this programme is not to arrange sporadic physical breast examinations of different kind made up by medical personnel, but to stimulate women themselves to regular and life-long BSE, checked by an efficient feed-back system.

On a national level the initiative for the programme can come from politicians, physicians, nurses, cancer organizations and individual women. Especially women's organizations can make an invaluable contribution by supporting the initiatives on different levels.

At the regional level, local politicians, physicians, nurses, universities, institutions and different organizations may also play a part, and cancer organizations can give support to different initiatives, as well as financial support.

At the local level, health personnel at places of work, employers and women on grass-root level can take the first step.

Many people realize already that the programme represents a longterm undertaking which cannot be kept going on a large scale in a country without some kind of response from society at large.

As long as the programme is kept intact as a multidimensional entity – person-to-person communication, feed-back and referral – variations in matters of detail should not diminish the programme's effect when implemented through different channels.

Target groups

There is much to be said for approaching women not in the vulnerable age group. Women should learn to know their own breasts while they are normal, e.g. at the age of 20 years. By regular BSE it will then be easier to recognize non malignant and malignant changes later on.

Thus in Finland an initiative has been taken by school nurses, starting the programme with pupils in the highest level. The girls have not only shown interest, but have contributed to take initiative themselves, often because their mothers participated in the test project. This shows that young women can indeed develop a positive attitude to the subject. The constructive health habit can then be adopted early, probably for life.

However, women need constant encouragement. Having left school, they can be reached through maternity counseling services for instance. Pregnant women as well can follow the programme. They can avoid the palpation phase of BSE but carry out the visual inspection even more carefully than usual. Women who are the target for public health check-ups (gynaecological check-ups, contraceptive counseling, post natal check-ups, etc.) can all be enrolled in the programme. Many women can be reached through the health-care facilities at their place of work – nearly 60 % of all adult women work in some industrialized countries outside their homes and have contact with some sort of health care at place of work. Adult women in older age groups – representing the highest risk groups for breast cancer – can be reached through women's organizations, pensioneers groups, gymnastic groups, etc. Such groups establish contact with a key-person who will carry through the programme either for a fee or on voluntary basis. And lastly, even previous breast cancer patients should for the rest of their lives go through with the programme. They can be encouraged to do so by the physicians in charge of their controls and other check-ups.

Many women who have themselves experienced the drawbacks of programmes for teaching the BSE technique only are very eager to support the multidimensional programme.

Key-persons

When information is to be conveyed in a BSE programme using person-to-person communication it is important that the task is carried out by people who actually know about breast cancer. The programme's informative element was therefore the responsibility of various nurses, physicians or their assistants, leaders of gymnastic groups and so on. In every case the credibility requirements call for some well trained person. But of course, these key-persons can also receive practical assistance from volunteers.

Clearly the most important steps at the various local levels are those taken by individual key-persons in making the programme part of their regular routine.

The key-persons inform the women and they act as a link between the ones with symptoms and the breast specialists. A person with a special strength of personality may be needed to pioneer the programme.

When speaking of the recruitment of key-persons, it might seem that most of the attention has been focused upon nurses. There are, however, many reasons for using physicians as key-persons, as well.

This programme would not disrupt any contact that a woman may already have with different doctors. On the contrary, all kinds of physicians can enrol women in this BSE-programme where they themselves assume the role of key-persons. And they can co-operate with breast specialists who are prepared to take the responsibility for the final diagnostic procedures to apply to those who are referred to them.

Such initiatives can come from physicians themselves who are interested in a continuous BSE-programme in the meantime between their own physical check-ups or examiniations with certain technical equipment.

Volunteers

As already emphasized, volunteers can plan and take initiatives at all levels, not least by making representations to political and medical decision makers. They can come forward from women's organizations, cancer organizations and other organizations. They can help to guarantee the continuity of the programme once it is established, by arranging for information meetings, distributing and collecting calendars, putting them in files, and giving reminders. They can be especially helpful, too, in counteracting fears and misunderstandings on person-to-person level about breast self-examination and the multidimensional programme.

Breast specialists

The specialists in this programme must be surgeons, radiologists, oncologists or cytologists.

At the start of the programme the breast specialists must be carefully told that the programme's long-term referral system should put very little pressure on them. The key-person and the volunteers do everything possible not only to help women who have detected symptoms themselves, but to prevent women without symptoms of breast cancer from requesting unneeded physicians consultations only because they are worried.

Breast specialists are often pleasantly surprised at the small workload entailed by the programme. Moreover, they want to help women who really need it.

Needless to say, the key-person and the specialist should preferably know each other well and have a good working relationship, for instance, if the breast specialist attends an information meeting, if only so as to hear in what terms his contribution to the programme is presented to the women.

Materials and money

In the beginning materials to train the key-persons are needed (this book) to help them prepare for their role, then for presentation overhead illustrations and the demonstration poster are required in addition to this book. In continuous programmes only the calendars are needed and inexpensive boxes for their collection.

The test project showed that the initial cost of the programme per woman reached was low as well as the cost per newly detected breast cancer case. Furthermore, the costs diminish in continuous programmes.

The cost for a breast specialist and the equipment aimed at consultation for women with self-detected symptoms will of course vary from country to country. But costs for the examination of women with symptoms only are very low in comparison to costs in connection with screenings, where asymptomatic women as well as symptomatic ones are to be examined, and the arrangements require special administration.

Similarly, the enrollment of key-persons does not represent any requirements for investment, since there are so many potential key-persons at various points within existing systems, which can carry through the programme within their daily routine.

Mass media

The media (TV, radio, the press, women's magazines, etc.) can alert decision-makers to the need for the programme and help to activate women to continuous breast self-examination activity. They can stress that the programme is not a short-term campaign but an incitement to a life-long behavioural pattern for every woman, and that it offers reassurance and protection in a cheap and simple way. All this will tend to create a climate of optimism.

The media should not limit themselves to BSE technique only, they should concentrate on: how the programme actually works and what it offers; cautious BSE technique and the importance of making BSE a permanent habit; and the importance of contacting the designated breast specialist if symptoms are detected by women themselves. And not the least service they can perform is in stressing the difference between the mass communication they themselves represent and the personalized communication system within the programme.

It means, of course, that the media people themselves must be carefully informed. They should be encouraged to read the literature on the subject so that a situation can never arise in which they and the programme's key-person are talking at cross purposes. It helps, too, if the medical personnel in the programme get to know the media people personally, so as to further co-operation.

In Finland mass media people have been informed by the present author about the programme as part of their training in certain centres. It has been gratifying to note how well they have grasped the programme's multidimensionality.

It is worth repeating, however, that mass media coverage is not permanently effective unless permanently maintained. During the test project period, for instance, one of the Finnish television channels transmitted the short spot film already mentioned. The main aim was to remind women in the project to keep on with BSE. But it had interesting side-effects as well.

Clearly, not all women can be encouraged to BSE on one and the same occasion. And a woman needs to be constantly reminded or re-encouraged through as many channels as possible. As the project showed, moreover, although most women respond best to person-to-person communication, for some women mass communication is important as a reminder. Mass media programmes are needed in order to remind decision-makers and key-persons also. Repetition is furthermore needed because every year the medical personnel will include new individuals in all public health functions. So the need for mass media coverage of the right kind is actually unremitting.

Summary and ideas for implementation

During recent decades breast cancer screening programmes have made valuable attempts to provide early breast cancer diagnosis. But screening is not the complete answer for the whole adult female population in any country. Screening can only be offered to certain groups of women. And repeated mammography should not be offered to women under 50 years.

For about 80 years women in many countries have been receiving information about breast cancer and breast self-examination. But the methods of information have not brought these abilities fully into play. Although women know about the desirability of monthly breast self-examination, they actually do very little.

What is needed is reassuring information which motivates women to perform monthly BSE, and to contact the proper physician. There has to be a real and uncomplicated link between every woman who detects breast cancer symptoms herself, and a breast specialist (surgeon, radiologist), and the key-person arranges for agreements with a breast specialist which will be selected for this very programme.

In this book a multidimensional programme for the early detection of breast cancer is described; the results of a test project and examples from the implementation of the programme in existing public health systems have been presented.

A few typical features of the programme are:
- Person-to-person communication;
  a medically trained key-person informs women about facts related to

breast self-examination and the actual programme aimed at early detection of breast cancer.

- A feed-back system;

    a special feed-back system and specially designed material is used in order to keep check on women's health behaviour regarding the regularity in breast self-examination.

- A specialist referral system;

    a direct link is established between women who detect breast cancer symptoms themselves and a breast specialist.

The breast self-examination technique used includes visual inspection and cautious palpation once a month according to exact instructions.

It was shown that the programme favourably changes women's attitudes; they feel no longer alone with their BSE. It changes health behaviour regarding breast self-examination; women perform BSE regularly, and this in its turn facilitates early diagnosis. The programme can be implemented in various systems and it could run with little cost continuously and on a broad scale, whereby it would play a major role in the struggle against breast cancer irrespective of the enrolled women's living area or socio-economic status.

The benefits of the multidimensional programme are given in the following table:

CONVENTIONAL HEALTH EDUCATION	THE MULTIDIMENSIONAL PROGRAMME
- mass communication efforts (brochures, films, articles) - personal instruction of BSE (one-way communication)	An entity of - person-to-person communication - feed-back system - referral to breast specialist
• DOES INCREASE KNOWLEDGE	• DOES INCREASE KNOWLEDGE
• DOES NOT ACCOMPLISH MONTHLY BSE	• DOES ACCOMPLISH MONTHLY BSE
• DOES NOT ENSURE CONTACT WITH BREAST SPECIALISTS	• DOES ENSURE CONTACT WITH BREAST SPECIALISTS
• SELDOM REDUCES PATIENT'S DELAY	• REDUCES PATIENT'S DELAY
• DOES NOT REDUCE DOCTOR'S DELAY	• REDUCES DOCTOR'S DELAY

An overview of the elements in the implementation of the multidimensional programme is given in the following table (based on the results of the test project):

IMPLEMENTATION OF THE BSE-CENTERED CONTINUOUS PROGRAMME IN DIFFERENT SYSTEMS

TARGET:	All women over 20 years disregarding living area
INITIATIVES:	Politicians Decision-makers Medical personnel Women's organizations Cancer organizations Women on grass root level
CHANNELS:	Schools Universities Public health centers General practitioner's offices Gynaecologist's offices Gynaecological screening centers Breast cancer screening centers
KEY-PERSONS:	Nurses General Practioners Family physicians Gynaecologists Other medical personnel
BREAST SPECIALISTS:	Surgeons Radiologists Oncologists Cytologists
MATERIAL:	The present book Overhead pictures Poster for demonstration Copies of calendars

Certain baseline data that are required when implementing the multidimensional systematic programme on a broad scale are given in the following table:

BASELINE DATA REGARDING A MODEL PROGRAMME FOR BREAST CANCER CONTROL IN A COUNTRY WITH 1 MILLION WOMEN AT RISK FOR BREAST CANCER, AND AN INCIDENCE OF 1 PER 1 000 WOMEN PER YEAR AND NORMALLY ABOUT 50 % OF THE CASES BEING EARLY ONES (estimate based on the results of the test project)

	FIRST YEAR	SECOND YEAR	YEARS FOLLOWING
Required N° of medical informants/key-persons*	1,000–10,000	1,000–10,000	1,000–10,000
Required N° of breast specialists*	50	50	50
N° of women receiving – information – calendar – link to breast specialist	1 Million	1 Million	1 Million
N° of women showing up with symptoms	10,000	<10,000	<10,000
N° of new breast cancer cases	1,800	700	1,000
Percentage early cases	70	>70	>70
Costs per new detected case in US $	200	<200	<200

* holding existing positions and devoting a small fraction of their daily work to their role in this programme

The present author's ideas regarding implementation of the Mama Programme in different health systems and recommendations on national, regional and local level have been discussed at conferences of the UICC (1974), the International Union for Health Education (1976, 1979), and on the Symposium for Prevention and Detection of Cancer (1976, 1980).

On the initiative of the Finnish women's organizations Marttaliitto and Finlands Svenska Marthaförbund (who initiated the project described in this book) one of the world's leading women's organizations, the Associated Country Women of the World, ACWW, has recommended the implementation of this programme on a world-wide scale in Recommendation No 2 in Nairobi 1977 and Recommendation Health 14 in Hamburg 1980.

References

Aarts, N.J.M.: The use of thermography in the detection of breast cancer. Bibl. Radiol. 5, 1969.

Ackerman, L.V.: The pathology of minimal breast carcinoma. The Swedish Cancer Society, Stockholm 1979.

Adlercreutz, H., Goldin, B.R., Dwyer, J.T., Warram, J.H., Gorbach, S.L.: Effect of diet on estrogen metabolism in women. J. Steroid. Biochemistry, 11:viii, 1979.

Alcoe, S., Butler, A.: A guide to breast self-examination. Canadian Cancer Society, New Brunswick Division, 1979.

Andersson, I.: Mammographic Screening for Breast Carcinoma. Malmö, 1980

Arner, O., Bergström,J., Franzén, S., Granberg, P-O., Rutqvist, L.E., Theve, N.O., Wallgren, A.: Delay in diagnosis of breast cancer. Läkartidningen, Sweden. Vol. 75, No 38, 1978.

Bailar, J.C.: Mammography, a contrary view. Ann. Int. Med. 84, 1976.

Beard, R.R.: Diagnostic screening tests. New Engl. J. Med. 275, 1966.

Cancer Incidence in Finland 1972. The Finnish Cancer Registry, Helsinki, Finland, 1975.

Collins, V.P., Loeffler, R.K., Tivey, H.: Observations on growth rates of human tumors. Am. J. Roentgenol. Radium. Ther. Nucl. Med., 1956.

Chamberlain, J.: Problems encountered in screening for breast cancer. UICC Techn. Report Ser. Vol. 40, 1978.

Clemmesen, J.: Bryst cancer. Statistiske forskningsresultater. Ugeskr. for laeger, 110, 1948.

Croll, J.: Mammography in Australia, M. J. Austr. 1, 1977.

De Saxe, B.M.: Breast at risk. S. Afr. Med. J., 47, 1973.

Duncan, W., Kerr, G.R.: The curability of breast cancer. Brit. Med. Journ. 2/10, 1976.

Elovainio, L.: Investigation on Health Education N° III. National Board of Health, Helsinki, Finland, 1980.

Elwood, J.M., Moorehead, W.P.: Delay in diagnosis and long-term survival in breast cancer. B. M. J., 31 May, 1980.

Gallager, H.S.: Developmental pathology of breast cancer. ACS, National Conference Breast Cancer, New York, 1979.

Gästrin, G., Ramström, L.: Smokingcessation, a challenge for medical personnel. Int. Journ. Health Education, Vol XVIII, No 1, 1975.

Gästrin, G.:
– Nordiska samarbetsmöjligheter i kampen mot bröstcancer. Nordisk Medicin, 88, 1973.
– Marttojen rintatutkimukset. Kampen mot Cancer 4, 1974 (Finl.).
– How education helps. World Health Magazine, November 1975.
– Mama-toiminta toivottuun päätökseen, Emäntälehti 11, 1976 (Finl.).
– Bröstcancerdiagnostik genom hälsofostran. Läkartidningen 73, 1976 (Swe).
– New technique for increasing the efficiency of self-examination in early diagnosis of breast cancer. B. M. J., October 1976.
– Terveyskasvatusohjelma rintasyöpäseulonnan apuna. Finlands Läkartidning 31, 1976.
– Uusi menetelmä rintasyövän toteamiseksi. Finlands Läkartidning 32, 1977.
– Egenvård för upptäckt av bröstcancer. Landstingens Tidskrift 8, 1977 (Swe).
– Tidig upptäckt av bröstcancer. Vigör 3, 1978 (Swe).
– Marttojen Mama-toiminnan tuloksia. Emäntälehti 1, 1979 (Finl).
– Tidig diagnostik av bröstcancer. Läkartidningen 41, 1979 (Swe).
– Mama-metoden – hälsoupplysningsmetod mot brönstcancer. Läkartidningen 77, 1980 (Swe).
– Programme to encourage self-examination for breast cancer. B. M. J. 197, 1980.
Gershon-Cohen, J.: Mammography. Wis. Med. Journ. 66, 1967.
Gyllensköld, K.: Visst blir man rädd. Forum, Sweden, 1976.
Gyllensköld, K.: Psychological aspects in connection with breast cancer information and diagnosis. The Swedish Cancer Society, Stockholm, 1979.

Hakulinen, T.: The Finnish Cancer Registry. Information by letter 1980.
Hallberg, O.: Breast Cancer Conference, Skövde, Sweden, Oct., 1979.
Haskell, C.M., Sparks, F.C., Thompson, R.W.: Breast Cancer. Cancer Treatment. W. B. Saunders Company, Philadelphia 1980.
Henderson, G., Canellos, G.P.: Cancer of the breast. The New Engl. Journ. of Medicine, Vol. 302, No 1, 1980.
Hill, D.J., Todd, P., Ryan, J., Magarey, C.J., Pickford, G., Lickiss, N., Hetzel, B.S., Krister, S.J.: Retrospective survey of women attending a hospital breast clinic. UICC Techn. Report Ser., Vol. 26, 1977.
Hillerdal, O.: Oral information, 1979.
Hinkamp, J.F.: The role of mammography in the diagnosis of breast cancer. Am. J. Obstet. Gynecol. III, 1971.
Hobbs, P., Haran, D.,Pendleton, L.: Breast screening by breast self-examination: An evaluation of teaching methods and materials. Dept. of Epidemiology and Social Research. University Hospital of South Manchester, 1980.
Holsti, L.: Institute of Radiotherapy, Helsinki: oral information 1980.

James, W.G.: Conduct of a public education programme. UICC Techn. Report Ser., Vol. 10, 1974.

Koulumies, M.: Cancer of the breast. Central Institute of Radiotherapy, Helsinki, 1956.

Lahti, R.: Applicability of clinical examination, mammography and thermography to mass screening for breast cancer. University of Turku, Finland, 1977.

Land, C.E.: Radiation – a cause of human breast cancer? ACS, National Conference Breast Cancer, New York, 1979.

Leis, Jr., H.P.: Presymptomatic diagnosis of breast cancer. Prog. Clin. Cancer, 4, 1970.

Lesnick, G.J.: Detection of breast cancer in young women. JAMA, March 7, 1977.

Lundgren, B.: Single oblique view mammography, an efficient method for breast cancer screening. Gävle, Sweden, 1980.

Lyyra, T.: Oral information, Helsinki, 1979.

Mäntylä, L.: Milloin rintasyöpää epäilevä nainen lähtee lääkääriin. CANCER No 6/The Finnish Cancer Society, Helsinki, 1980.

Mustakallio, S.: Conservative treatment of breast carcinoma. Clin. Radiolog. 23, 1972.

Nordenström, B.: Stereotactic fine-needle biopsy in connection with mammography. Läkartidningen, Sweden, Vol. 76/23, 1979.

Räf, L.: Early diagnosis in breast cancer. Läkartidningen, Sweden, 41, 1979.

Räsänen, O., Auranen, A., Grönroos, M.: Two years experience about breast cancer screening and health information in Turku 1977–1978. The Swedish Cancer Society. Stockholm, 1979.

Selvini, A.: Delay in diagnosis due to the patient. Publ. Educat. Cancer, 11, 1974.

Serén, M.: Statistics of Marthas, Turku Region. Oral information 1981.

Shapiro, S., Strax, P., Venet, L.T.: Evaluation of periodic breast cancer screening with mammography. JAMA 195, 1966.

Shapiro, S.: Efficacy of breast cancer screening. UICC Techn. Report Ser., Vol. 40, 1978.

Soini, I.: Risk factors and selective screening for breast cancer. University of Tampere, Finland, 1977.

Standerskjöld-Nordenstam, C-G., Svinhufvud, U.: Mammography of symptomatic breasts. Ann. Chir. Gyn. II, Vol. 69, 1980.

Stewens, G.M.: Variations and supplementary techniques in mammography. Oncology, 23, 1969.

Strax, P.: Does annual mammography help? Int. Sympos. on Detection of Breast Cancer. Copenhagen, 1977.

Strax, P.: Long term results of H.I.P. mass screening program for breast cancer. Fourth International Symposium on the Detection of Cancer, London, 1980.

Teppo, L., Hakulinen, T., Saxén, E.: Prediction of the cancer incidence in Finlnd in 1980. Duodecim 89, 1973.

Teppo, L., Hakama, M., Hakulinen, T., Lehtonen, M., Saxén, E.: Cancer in Finland 1953–1970: Incidence, Mortality, Prevalence. Acta Pathologica et Mikrobiologica Scandinavica, Sect. A, 1975.

83

The Gallup Organization, Conducted for the ACS: Women's attitudes regarding breast cancer. New York, 1976.

Venet, L.: Self-examination and clinical examination of the breast. ACS, National Conference Breast Cancer, New York, 1979.

Verres, R.: Psychologic aspects in planning preventive care operations. Georg Thieme Verlag, Stuttgart, 1978.

Wakefield, J.: Measurement and evaluation. UICC Techn. Report Ser., Vol. 10,1974.

Wallace, D.: Self help in the detection of breast cancer. 10th Internat. Conference on Health Education, London, 1979.

Appendix

Manual for key-persons

Running the programme

The task of people involved

Decision-makers

Concerned individuals, women's organizations, cancer societies and others should arrange for information about the multidimensional, systematic and continuous programme and its potentialities to reach politicians and other decision-makers who will be in the position to promote the implementation of the multidimensional programme in different health systems and in different contexts.

The people who implement this programme in existing health systems should arrange for financing the programme. The costs will be for the manual and the eventual salary for the key-person, for the hire of a room where the information meeting takes place and for the calendars for every woman every year. In places of work, working hours should be used for information purposes. This is a limited expense compared to the benefit of early detection in one of the employees.

The people who make the decision of implementing this multidimensional programme in existing health care systems should arrange supplies of the materials needed:

For decision-makers and medical personnel: the present book.

For the key-persons: the present book as a manual, overhead illustrations and the poster for demonstration.

For the breast specialists: a notebook or file records on women who will show up with symptoms.

For volunteers: the poster for reminding purposes.

For mass media: correct descriptions given by decision makers and medical staff.

For participating women: a new calendar each year, which is given to them in connection with the personal instruction.

Breast specialists

In different public health systems the link to the breast specialist must be established before the information meetings for the women are arranged. The breast specialist in every programme can be invited to attend an information meeting and should take part in the discussion with the women in the programme. Sometimes it is arranged that the women who detect symptoms themselves first contact they key-person. But the breast specialist should in any case be the final instance, and the breast specialists must be informed in advance how many women will show up at their offices. This is easy to predict in every programme to be planned because of the results in the project described in this book. Each year about 1 % of those women who get information and a calendar will show up at the breast specialist's office. If the programme does not work under optimal circumstances maybe 5 % per year of those who received information and a calendar will show up.

The breast specialists should take care of, and keep records on, women who show up with self-detected symptoms as a result of the multidimensional programme.

Key-persons

Nurses, physicians (general practitioners/family physicians, gynaecologists, etc. for example in charge of breast physical examinations, mammograms, and other check-ups), medical assistants, should:
- arrange for person-to-person communication with individual women or women in groups;
- arrange the link with a particular breast specialist;
- get together the materials needed by key-persons and the women who are to be target of the programme;
- give person-to-person information about cautious BSE technique and the multidimensional programme;
- give every woman a calendar and the name of the breast specialist she can turn to. The initial distribution of calendars should only take place in connection to personal contact between the key-persons/volunteers and the women thereby being enrolled in the programme;
- collect the calendars at the end of every year, put them in files, and issue new ones;
- arrange co-operation with the mass media for the purposes of activating and reminding other key-persons and women to continue with the programme.

Volunteers

Within different public health systems and functions, places of work, schools, women's and other organizations, there are volunteers who could: help with arrangements for individual counseling or for meetings, with distributing, collecting and filing the calendars, handing out new ones every year, with shaping attitudes through person-to-person interface and with giving relevant information about local projects to mass media representatives.

PEOPLE IN THE MAMA PROGRAMME

Gästrin 1981

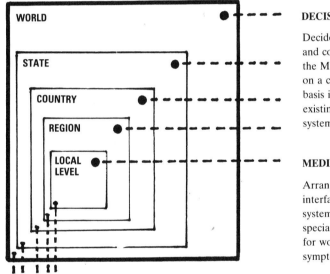

| WORLD | ● ← ─ ─ ─ | **DECISION MAKERS** |

Decide, implement and coordinate the Mama Programme on a continuous basis in existing health systems

MEDICAL STAFF

Arrange for person-to-person interface, the feed-back system, and the breast specialist referral system for women who detect symptoms

All women can be enrolled in a Mama Programme on **all levels** and with continuity

Manual for the information meeting

Preparations

Information meetings within the health services at places of work should take place during working hours. For groups of students in schools and high schools, colleges and universities, and for women in organizations and gymnastic groups, pensioneers, and in different public health functions the information could take place after working hours.

A meeting, including question-time, should take about one hour. It sometimes happens that not all women will actually want to join the programme at the first meeting. Sometimes, for practical reasons, all women are not able to attend the first information meeting. The meeting should be arranged well in advance so that the women are given plenty of time. If a great number of women seem unable to attend then, a second meeting should also be arranged. Sometimes women can influence each other on the basis of group interaction, and when a new meeting is arranged most of the women will want to attend. No woman can be forced to join the programme.

The best size for a meeting is between 20 and 50 women; in a larger group discussion is more difficult. It is important, too, that the atmosphere at the meeting should be informal and relaxed.

The room in which the meeting takes place should be suitable for showing pictures in darkness or semi-darkness (depending on the apparatus used) and have good lighting for when the key-person demonstrates BSE-techniques on herself or writes down figures on the blackboard.

Person-to-person information need not always happen in groups. In certain contexts it is possible for the key-person to give information to individuals. In such situations it will not take a whole hour to explain background factors and the new communication strategy and to demonstrate cautious BSE technique on the woman herself.

The course of the meeting

General remarks

Before the key-person starts giving information it is advisable to do a target group analysis, so that the information can be adapted to different kinds of receptivity. Obviously groups can be either homogenous or heterogenous in structure. To no small extent the key-person will have to rely on her own experience and intuition to help her establish contact with different people.

Before the key-person has become used to conducting meetings, she may find it helpful to have still plainer guidelines to follow during the discussion and the lecture phases of the meeting. A specimen lecture is therefore printed below, together with the guidelines for discussion.

These can be adapted for various circumstances though the structure of discussion:

– Background information to reassure and motivate.

This should create a feeling of security and arouse the women's sense of responsibility for their own well-being. The information should be in no way sensationalistic. Breast cancer should be discussed as one of many other problems in a person's life.

– A description of the multidimensional communication strategy of the breast cancer control programme described in this book. One can mention the 56 177 women in the test-project in Finland. The aim was to test person-to-person communication with a feed-back system and a pre-arranged referral system. The method is not based on mass communication, like the distribution of brochures, even though the cautious BSE technique can also be read about in brochures. One can mention and decribe parts of the evaluated project and write down figures regarding the project results. The message has of course to be adapted to the target group in question.

– A detailed description of cautious BSE technique.

A main aim here is to guard against dangerous techniques such as massage and careless finger-tip palpation. Cautious BSE technique consist of visual inspection and gentle palpation.

– An exact description of the referral system to the breast specialist in charge of women who detect breast cancer symptoms themselves.

The information must of course be adjusted to the situation and expectations of the women listening. Some women want to know the worst about breast cancer. They should be frankly told, though with a reminder that if women are active on their own behalf the prognosis will be much better. It is important, too, to give ample information, so that women feel that they are really well placed to make a decision about regular BSE. Factual information and serious discussion in groups or with individuals will motivate most women.

Opening discussion

The key-person can start the meeting by welcoming those attending and thanking the people who have arranged it, and she should try to create a relaxed atmosphere straight away. She can say that a question time will follow her lecture, and that time can be saved if all the information can be given in one go, but she should not be surprised if questions are asked before the question-time proper.

An information meeting can start with a discussion. This demands considerable flexibility on the part of the key-person, and therefore it is important that the key-person has a sound medical background.

Women who have received full and reassuring information can positively influence each other in group interaction just as smokers do in smoking cessation programmes. Most women *know* that they ought to examine their breasts. So one can ask the women at the meeting how many already do so once a month. Then the question of fear – fear of the disease itself and fear of information about it – can be taken up. And here it is important to emphasize considerations which can give a sense of security, and the reasons for the personalized attention now being offered. One can mention the kind of information that has been given previously. Most women are rather surprised when they realize that the information now being offered is connected with a feed-back system – the calendars. The general point should also be stressed that the aim of the programme is to change health behaviour *for life*. It is not a short-term campaign and it is not a medical check-up. Every woman should learn to know *her own* breasts as each woman's breasts *are unique*.

One can also mention the different techniques of BSE, and stress that the programme is based on the cautious method. In fact the programme avoids everything that could cause either physical or psychological harm.

A specimen lecture: text and illustrations

There is not just one type of cancer. – Cancer varies depending on which organ of the body is affected, age, and other circumstances.

Some cancer diseases can be prevented by what is called primary prevention. That is to say, the very cause of the disease can be removed. This is the case with smoker's lung cancer, which can be prevented by not smoking.

Many other cancer diseases cannot be primarily prevented. Only secondary prevention is possible, which is as much as to say early diagnosis. One such disease is breast cancer which is the most common cancer in women after the age of 30 years.

The breast cancer figures have increased slowly in most countries during the last two decades in all age groups, but survival rates have been influenced only very little. The risk factors which do seem to play an

92

important part are: an age over 30; nulliparity, late age at first pregnancy, a history of breast cancer in close relatives (though breast cancer is not hereditary). But a discussion of risk factors, though of theoretical interest, gives little practical guidance. A woman who has all the known risk factors may not get breast cancer, and a woman with none of them may.

Breast cancer seems to be different in different women.

Some breast cancer cases may have a slow growth while others grow rapidly, some extremly rapidly. Therefore in all breast cancers there is a need for a frequent search programme.

Medical treatment is constantly developing as women report their symptoms earlier; more and more women can be offered the chance of limited breast cancer surgery, different kind of reconstruction of a breast, etc, which earlier did not exist at all. Of course this does not mean that limited surgery already can be offered to all patients yet. But every breast cancer patient should have these opportunities. Even if the idea of breast cancer is very alarming at first, every woman who actually gets it will be grateful for being an early diagnosed case.

Not only the quality of life is influenced by early diagnosis and limited surgery; also life expectancy changes totally if a woman is treated early, from the situation if she is treated at a late stage.

Most people know from medical reports and from mass media information that there are screening programmes for breast cancer as well as there are screening programmes for the early detection of cervical cancer (Pap tests). Breast cancer screenings are offered to certain groups of women in certain parts of some countries. Most well known are screenings for breast cancer with mammography technique. But this type of screening simply is not available to most women and repeated exposure to radiation may result in harm to young women's breasts. Still today there is no medical screening technique which is safe, frequent enough and offered to all women in the world. But screening tests have shown that *something* can be done in order to detect early breast cancers and in offering early treatment. This is the most hopeful message that can be given to all women.

When it comes to all women of the world the only really frequent control of the breasts is by monthly regular breast self-examination; as already underlined, breast cancer symptoms *can* occur very rapidly.

We have known for a long time that women themselves are excellent what comes to detection of symptoms of breast cancer. Of those women who are registered as new breast cancer patients, 90 % first detected the symptoms of breast cancer themselves. However, in most cases the self-detection is by accident only and women do not immediately show up at a breast specialist's consultation. This calls for a more systematic programme for breast cancer control, using the women's own ability in BSE. If women learn to know their own breasts while they are still healthy they can learn what is normal and thus there will be good chances to detect symptoms of breast cancer even at an early stage. Women are able to detect both non-malignant and malignant symptoms in their breasts themselves by breast self-examination. Women who start performing regular monthly breast self-examination while their breasts are healthy can recognize non malignant changes in connection with menstruation; with pregnancy and breast feeding; with increasing age, etc. It is to be remembered that more than 95 % of all changes from what is normal in women's breasts are *not* breast cancer symptoms; less than 5 % of all breast changes that are detected by the women themselves are caused by breast cancer. Women who know their own breasts posess the capability to detect malignant changes as well, as will be described later in connection with a showing of pictures.

Descriptions of breast self-examination technique and what to look for sometimes contradict each other. Some informants recommend the cautious BSE technique while others recommend massage of the breasts with the finger-tips.

Because some studies suggest that injuries may be one of the reason for the development of breast cancer, the only safe way to perform breast self-examination is visual inspection (looking) and cautious palpation (feeling). The best time for examining the breasts is immediately after menstruation when the breasts are soft and not tender to touch. Regular breast self-examination is therefore recommended every month immediatcly after periods. Women who have no periods should examine their breasts once a month as well.

But how shall women be motivated to perform regular monthly breast self-examination?

Mass communication efforts like brochures, films, articles in women's magazines, etc, can influence knowledge about the desirability of breast self-examination. But women's fears and anxiety about breast cancer have long been played on for sensationalistic purposes through mass communication. Women are often worried because they do not know exactly which breast self-examination technique they shall use; they do not know exactly what to look for; they cannot discuss questions in a factual way; and they do not know which physician to see if symptoms occur. This makes women passive even if they are aware of the problem.

94

Person-to-person communication by a person who is trustworthy is more effective than mass communication when it comes to influencing people's behaviour, e.g. their health behaviour regarding regular breast self-examination; women can question the informant about BSE, about the BSE-technique, what exactly to look for, their individual problems, and what to do if symptoms occur.

One special comprehensive, systematic type of breast cancer control programme has been tested in a large test-project with 56 000 women enrolled. This programme was based on the followng principles:
– Person-to-person information on breast self-examination including discussions
– A feed-back system for monthly regular and life long continuous BSE
– A breast specialist selected in advance to take care of those women who were to detect symptoms of breast cancer themselves when performing monthly breast self-examination

It was shown that the fears women felt in the beginning changed into a positive concern, and the women were then motivated to perform regular BSE every month, and they showed up at the pre-arranged breast specialist's office if they detected breast cancer symptoms. Thousands of women have experienced the same effect since the test-project ended and the method has been implemented in existing public health functions.

In Finland medical staff, supported by decision-makers, women's organizations and active individual women have already arranged for continuous and geographically complete programmes and these programmes can year by year and step by step cover a whole population, irrespective of who the women are and where they live. Breast self-examination should be a life-long habit for every woman and enable early breast cancer diagnosis to every woman in large population groups.

The main aim of the programme is to encourage women to learn to know their own breasts. In connection with the information, individual women's breasts can be physically examined in order to serve as something like a baseline check-up. However, such a physical examination gives the individual woman a false feeling of security that *something* has been done.

Most women are offered neither breast physical examination (e.g. in connection with their yearly gynaecological check-up, or with their Pap-test every three or five years) nor breast examinations in connection with breast cancer screenings at exactly the time when they become breast cancer patients. Physician's check-ups (from the individual woman's point of view sporadic) must be complemented with a systematic, regular, life-long programme for the early diagnosis of every growing breast cancer. Breast self-examination constitutes such a programme if performed in a continuous, systematic way. The system has to include immediate referral to a breast specialist for clinical diagnosis if a woman has detected symptoms of breast cancer herself.

In order to "catch" breast cancer cases at an early stage, women over 20 years of age should begin breast self-examination regularly on a monthly basis to learn to know their own breasts when still healthy and they should show up at a breast specialist's office immediately if they detect any symptom of breast cancer. And women who are uncertain about their findings when performing BSE should show up at the breast specialist's office too.

Breast self-examination should become the basic programme for early detection of breast cancer.

In this programme every woman will be offered:
- Encouragement to perform monthly cautious BSE
- A copy of a calendar for regular notes
- Information about the name ofthe breast specialist whom to consult immediately if any symptom(s) occur.

Written material which reminds on: breast self-examination technique, what to look for, and the name of the breast specialist who is selected in advance, will be distributed at the end of the information meeting with groups, or at the end of the information to individual women after the demonstration and discussion. There is no need for writing down details that are explained in the lecture or in connection with individual instruction. Everyone should just relax, hear and look.

In order to make things clear illustrations for demonstration purposes have been prepared and comments will be given. When the question-time starts further problems can be discussed.

A NORMAL BREAST IN A WOMAN OF ABOUT 20 YEARS

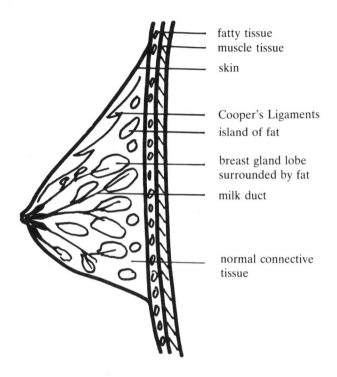

fatty tissue
muscle tissue

skin

Cooper's Ligaments
island of fat

breast gland lobe
surrounded by fat

milk duct

normal connective
tissue

COMMENTARY TO ILLUSTRATION 1/7:

This illustration shows a normal young woman's breast. The breast is consti-
tuted of ten to twenty breast gland lobes, each one ending in milk ducts, which
end in the nipple. The breast gland lobes together with islands of fatty tissue give
a firm and homogenous structure to the breast. Superficial so called Cooper's
ligaments give the shape to the breast.

The borders of the lobes in the breast tissue can sometimes be felt with the
fingers. If there is much fatty tissue in the breast, the borders mostly cannot be
felt. Before menstruation a feeling of fullness and tenderness of the breasts is
common.

Ideally all women should learn to know their own breasts by looking and
feeling before and after menstruation already at about 20 years of age while
everyone can learn what is normal for herself. This could make it easy to notice
any changes, would such later occur. The habit of monthly regular BSE should
start at this very age, but most women start later on.

ILLUSTRATION 2/7, The Mama Programme by Gisela Gästrin © 1981
THE BREASTS BETWEEN 25 AND 50 YEARS OF AGE

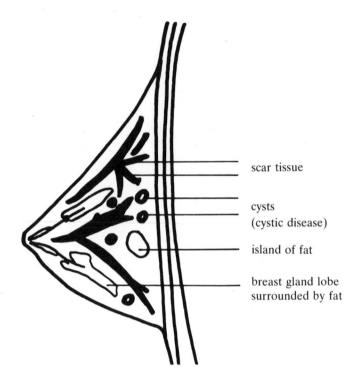

scar tissue

cysts
(cystic disease)

island of fat

breast gland lobe
surrounded by fat

COMMENTARY TO ILLUSTRATION 2/7:
Between the ages of 25 and 50 years and after pregnancies there can be a considerable amount of changes to the different tissues in the breasts. Changes in the connective tissue can be compared to scar tissue, and single or multiple cavities, called cysts, form together so called "cystic disease", being non malignant changes in the breasts of most adult women. The cysts are filled with body fluid or blood. Before menstruation the cysts are filled with more fluid than after menstruation; consequently the cysts feel hard before menstruation. In order to avoid wrong conclusions when performing breast self-examination, it is important to palpate the breasts immediately *after menstruation* when the cysts feel soft at palpation. Lumps that come and go with the menstrual period are most often non malignant while lumps that persist throughout the whole menstruation period of one month may be a sign of breast cancer.

After the age of 50 years the cysts often disappear and the breasts consist mainly of fatty tissue.

At the ages of 25–50 it is urgent for every woman to learn what is "normal" for her, thus enabling the self detection of abnormal findings, would such later occur.

ILLUSTRATION 3/7, The Mama Programme by Gisela Gästrin © 1981
BREAST SELF-EXAMINATION TECHNIQUE
First step: Visual inspection (looking)

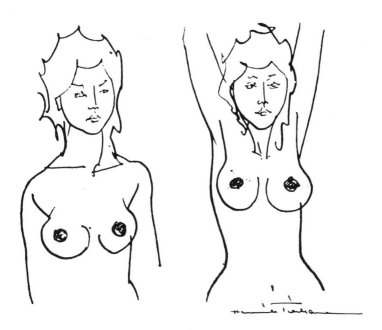

COMMENTARY TO ILLUSTRATION 3/7:

Stand in front of a mirror in good light. The inspection should be carried out once with the arms hanging down in a natural position, and once with the arms stretched up above your head. Turn your chest slightly to the right and then to the left so as to see both breasts from different angles. If your breasts are large, you can use your hands to help you see their undersides. Through regular BSE you will learn *what is normal for you.*

Breast cancer symptoms that you can detect by self-inspection are:
- Unequal elevation
- Increase or decrease in size
- Retraction of the skin
- Orange coloured skin
- Assymmetry of nipples
- Retraction of one nipple
- The nipple is sore
- Bloody discharge from the nipple

If you find one or more of these symptoms, or if you are uncertain about your finding, then contact the key-person or the breast specialist in this programme at once.

99

ILLUSTRATION 4/7, The Mama Programme by Gisela Gästrin © 1981
BREAST SELF-EXAMINATION TECHNIQUE
Second step: Cautious palpation (feeling)

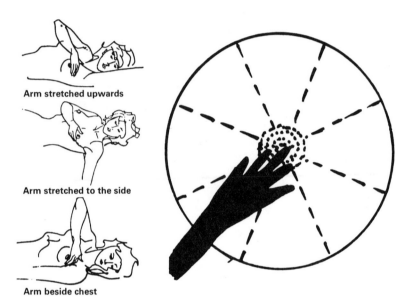

Arm stretched upwards

Arm stretched to the side

Arm beside chest

COMMENTARY TO ILLUSTRATION 4/7:

Lie down so that the breast to be examined is as flat as possible on the chest wall. A small pillow can be put under the shoulder on the side to be examined. Soap or creme-lotion can be used so as to make the skin slippery for gentle palpation. Use the opposite hand for palpation and palpate both breasts carefully.

With the palm and the whole length of the fingers cautiously press the breast against the chest wall sector by sector. Always lift the palpating hand, as you move from one sector to the next. Avoid any kind of massage or rough touching with the finger-tips.

Palpation of the whole breast should be performed three times, as shown in the picture: with the arm of the side to be examined placed first upwards, then to the side and lastly beside the chest.

Always palpate your breasts after menstruation. If you have no menstruations, you should still examine your breasts once a month. During pregnancy and breast feeding do not palpate your breasts – make only the visual inspection.

By palpation there can be found both non-malignant and malignant changes from normal. If a woman knows what is normal for her, she will be able to notice changes from normal, both non malignant, and malignant ones.

100

NON MALIGNANT CHANGES IN THE BREASTS
THAT ARE SELF-DETECTABLE THROUGH PALPATION

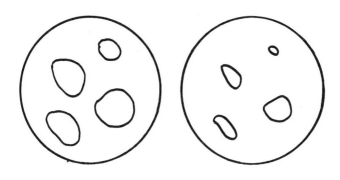

Cysts before menstruation   *Cysts after menstruation*

COMMENTARY TO ILLUSTRATION 5/7:

Non malignant changes in women's breasts after the age of 25 years are most often diagnosed as "cystic disease of the breast". Thus the breast tissue partly changes forming cavities of different size. As already described the cysts are before menstruation filled with more fluid than after menstruation. Before menstruation these cysts feel large, hard and are tender – a typical sign for non malignant changes of a breast. After menstruation the cysts feel small, soft and are not tender. If these typical benign changes are noticed by a woman herself, there is no reason for immediate consultation with the physician selected in advance in the Mama Programme.

If changes persist throughout the menstruation period, the breast specialist should be contacted immediately.

If a woman feels uncertainty the breast specialist should be contacted, as well.

There are some rare changes in the breast tissue, which are first non malignant and later may become breast cancer. Therefore all self-suspicions should be shown to the breast specialist.

MALIGNANT CHANGES IN THE BREASTS
THAT ARE SELF-DETECTABLE THROUGH PALPATION

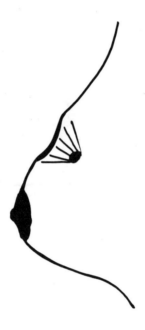

COMMENTARY TO ILLUSTRATION 6/7:

.Breast cancer symptoms that you can detect by palpation are:
- A lump in the breast or a hard mass, that does not disappear after menstruation, that persists in size or grows from one monthly palpation to the next.
Often a breast cancer lump is not really as large as it seems: the malign tumour
is often surrounded by connective tissue. Sometimes there will be a retraction
of the skin over the cancer lump.
- Sometimes, but not always pain in connection to palpation after monthly
menstruation may disclose a breast cancer. This sign may also exist in older
women without menstruations.
If you detect a lump that is hard and clearly different from other breast tissue
or cystic changes, the breast specialist should be contacted immediately.

ILLUSTRATION 7/7, The Mama Programme by Gisela Gästrin © 1981

BREAST CANCER CONTROL FROM THE WOMAN'S POINT OF VIEW

		Clinical detection quality	Geographical completeness	Continuity
SCREENING	with mammography	+	−	−
	by other methods	−	−	−
BREAST PHYSICAL EXAMINA-TION	non-breast specialist	(+)	−	−
	breast specialist	+	−	−
BREAST SELF-EXAMINA-TION	*SPORADIC* after isolated teaching of BSE	(+)	−	−
	SYSTEMATIC by enrollment in Mama Programme	+	+	+

VALUE: + high □ □ (+) satisfactory □ □ − poor

COMMENTARY TO ILLUSTRATION 7/7:

Too many breast cancers are allowed to grow until they are severe enough to be noticed by *accidental observation* by the woman herself. Since this is an utterly unsatisfactory situation there is a need for *active procedures* for early detection, i.e. breast cancer control activities. This illustration gives an overview of possible methods for breast cancer control.

Much is being done to improve clinical diagnostic methods, equipment and administration (screenings for example).

Physicians are being offered special education aimed at improving their overall knowledge and interest in breast diseases (breast physical examination).

But screening and breast physical examination are not offered to all women at the time when they become breast cancer patients.

In order to develop a continuous search for breast cancer the central role is played by individual women. Women possess the capability to detect breast cancer symptoms. This is presupposed by BSE-centered programmes (health education).

103

Sporadic teaching of BSE by itself does not constitute a good activation method for regular and continuous BSE.

A systematic BSE Programme including
- personal instruction
- a feed back system
- a breast specialist referral system

is a continuous one and offers high quality clinical detection. It can be offered to women on a worldwide scale. The Mama Programme fulfils these requirements.

Question-time

If it is difficult to get a discussion going after the lecture the key-person herself can ask some questions:
- Did this information make you feel more apprehensive or more secure?
- Do you feel motivated to start the programme immediately?
- Can you arrange practical details in your home for the purposes of BSE? Is there a mirror that you can stand in front of in a room with good lighting?

It is worthwhile to let women discuss their ideas among themselves so as to develop group dynamics.

It is important to keep a tight rein on the discussion. Individual woman's problems or earlier sufferings from cancer need not be discussed at length. If somebody does say they have a symptom like those described in the lecture, she should be advised to contact the programme's breast specialist at once.

If somebody wants a comparison of the information strategy of brochures with that of person-to-person communication, it should be mentioned that the two complement each other. The important thing is that they both describe *cautious* BSE technique. Thanks to brochures, women have *known* about breast cancer for a long time. Now it is time to *do* something about it.

The key-person should not be surprised if she gets some questions that she cannot answer. She should frankly admit her limitations, and promise to find out the answer as soon as she can. However, some questions are almost certain to come up, and for these she can be prepared:

Question: Is it necessary to examine the armpits?

Answer: In the information given no mention has been made of the armpits and how to examine them. It is often rather difficult for women to examine their armpits themselves and to differ between lumps of different origin. Many people quite normally have nodes which could arouse unnecessary concern in connection with BSE.

Breast cancer always starts in the breasts, and the most important thing is to get to know your breasts. If symptoms occur, then the specialist will also check the armpits.

Question: If a woman has the risk factors mentioned, what are the chances that she actually will get breast cancer?

Answer: There is no simple answer. A woman with many risk factors may never get the disease. A woman with none may. Either way, it is essential to perform regular BSE.

Question: How old should you be when you start the programme?

Answer: If you get to know your breasts when they are healthy you have a better chance of detecting any changes. The best age is therefore about 20.

Needless to say, though, if somebody is older than 20 and has not yet started, she should in any case start at once and go on for the rest of her life.

Question: What about contraceptive pills and the hormones that are used during menopause? Do they in any way tend to make breast cancer more likely?

Answer: This has not so far been proved, at least as far as contraceptives are concerned. On the other hand, if women do use hormones during menopause they are already in great breast cancer risk because of their age. They should discuss with their gynaecologist whether they should use hormones or not. If breast cancer has already occured no hormones should be used unless recommended by an oncologist.

Question: Do earlier breast problems – inflammations, injuries, abscesses, trauma, etc. – tend to make breast cancer more likely?

Answer: There are certain changes in the breast that *can* precede cancer, but of course not always. Sometimes there are hard lumps or scaring after an abscess, or surgery, etc. If you already know about hard lumps, or if you find some after this meeting, you should contact the programme's specialist at once, since breast cancer can also be a hard lump. The whole point of this programme is to bring breast cancer symptoms to light.

Question: Should pregnant women join the programme?

Answer: During pregnancy and the early period of breast feeding the breasts are tender. They should not be palpated. But the usual visual inspection should be carried out thoroughly and regularly. So there is no pause in the programme.

Question: Should women who have had breast cancer earlier join the programme?

Answer: Sometimes, though very seldom, breast cancer can occur in the opposite breast after one breast has been removed. Therefore, previous patients should inspect and palpate the remaining breast carefully.

Question: Why are som patients treated differently than others?

Answer: It mainly depends on how soon the woman consults a specialist. The treatment has to be tailor-made to suit the stage of development reached by the disease. The sooner a woman presents her symptoms the better, since then surgery can be less radical – limited surgery has been used in early detected cases and radiotherapy does not always have to be used.

Closing discussion

Immediately in connection with the question-time the key-person can start the closing discussion. She may add some remarks about changes that may take place in a woman's breasts apart from breast cancer; e.g. old women or women with large breasts, or hanging breasts (after many pregnancies), often find the sides of their breasts tender. This is not a sign of breast cancer. For several weeks they should wear a bra at night, and keep the breasts warm. Needless to say, though, these women can of course get breast cancer just like anybody else, and should perform regular monthly breast self-examination.

What is offered in this programme is a sense of security, and rapid attention should it be necessary, so there is no need to think about breast cancer all the time. Just remember breast self-examination once a month, straight after the monthly menstruation.

Breast self-examination is easy to learn. With increasing skill it will take only a few minues every month.

And once more: most changes from what is normal for a woman are not symptoms of breast cancer. There is no need to be worried because of every symptom, but instead to be concerned and aware of all the favourable possibilities in connection with self-care.

Therefore this programme has been developed. Every women in this programme receives exact instructions about who is the breast specialist in charge and how he/she should be contacted if symptoms are detected.

If the breast specialist of the actual programme has attended the information meeting where the key-person gave the information and the practical instructions, the breast specialist may introduce himself/herself during the information meeting.

During the last part of the closing discussion the key-person can herself once more demonstrate how to stand for the visual inspection and how to lie down for the palpation of first one and then the other breast.

It is particularly important to show how to ensure that the palpation is cautious. She can show how the whole hand, palm and the whole length of the fingers which are held close together, presses the breast gland in a cautious way sector by sector against the chest wall, and how the hand must be lifted as it moves from one sector to the next. No massage-like movements should be made. The key-person can show on her own breast how never to use the finger-tips and she can describe that regular incautious handling of the breasts can be dangerous because the breast is a very sensitive organ.

At an information meeting the key-person should carefully explain why she does *not* examine individual women's breasts: The women might receive the false impression that it is a question of a screening procedure. The responsibility for breast cancer diagnosis can never rest on an individual key-person during a single occasion. A woman can get breast cancer at some time when there is nobody to examine her, and therefore it is wrong to encourage a sense of security based only on the fact that *something* was done once. The point is to motivate every woman to get to know her breasts *herself* so that then, in carrying out regular BSE, she will easily be able to notice any changes that may occur.

Handing out the calendars

When the opening discussion, the lecture, question-time and the closing discussion have come to an end, the calendars should be handed out. It should then be stressed again that the calendar contains: a summary of BSE technique a space for notes about regular monthly BSE; and the name of the breast specialist in the programme to be consulted immediately if symptoms occur. The breast specialist's name should be written by the key-person on the calendars before they are distributed. The name of the breast specialist or some "contact person", can be filled in, if a programme differs at that very point, from the test-project.

When handing out the calendars, it is advisable to repeat how they are to be *filled in, returned* and *renewed each year.* Their generative function should also be stressed:

1. The woman is not left on her own. She can contact the key-person if she wants to know something, and she can contact the breast specialist if she finds a breast cancer symptom. And the calendar in which the name of the breast specialist is written down, will help her do so.

2. The calendar is a device enabling the key-person to see if the message has been understood and acted upon. And this check is continuous if the calendar is renewed every year.

When the calendars are handed out the women can be reminded that the calendar is a means of communication between them and the key-person. The same key-person or an assistant will after one year hand out new calendars, and collect the old ones.

When the new calendars are exchanged for the old ones, it is a good idea to check that the women have understood the message, and of course to tell them about any changes that may have occurred in the specialist referral system.

Person-to-person communication should preferably be continuously repeated if possible. Then a woman who forgets to ask an important question on one occasion, or who only thinks of it afterwards, can ask next time. Furthermore, the effect of the message can be cumulative. A woman feels more and more inclined to take advice offered, even if only to show that she appreciates the concern that is being shown for her well-being.

In connection with the exchange of calendars every year the message to women in a continuous Mama Programme can be repeated:
– The person-to-person information on breast self-examination
– The feed-back system for monthly regular, systematic and life-long BSE (the calendar-system)
– The name and address of the breast specialist selected in advance for those women who detect any breast cancer symptom(s), always to be written down in the new calendar each year.

Repetition of the message to women in a continuous Mama Programme in connection with the yearly exchange of calendars:

Mammography, ultrasound, cytology, etc. are used in high quality breast cancer detection programmes for the detection of early breast cancer. These diagnostic procedures are favourable in those cases only, when the females, who are offered examination at the time of the actual examination have breast cancer.

Breast physical examination which is performed systematically by medical personnel is favourable in those cases only, when the women who are offered physical examination, have breast cancer at the very time of this examination.

Breast self-examination has shown to be of great value, because women possess the capability to detect symptoms of breast cancer themselves, and then show up at breast specialist's consultations if symptoms occur.

It is a fact that most of the women in the world are never offered high level technical examinations or breast physical examination at physician's offices at the time-point when their breast cancer grows. This is the case both at physician's consultations and in connection with screenings for breast cancer. These examinations, which are sporadic from the women's point of view may give a false sense of security to women, that *something* has been done (all women who are offered sporadic examinations should of course take advantage of it and in connection with the examinations ask about involvment in a systematic and continuous breast self-examination programme).

The only way to achieve *frequent enough examination* for early detection of breast cancer symptoms is by regular *breast self-examination*. And BSE is performed frequent enough only if performed monthly.

It has been shown that isolated teaching of BSE-technique does *NOT* influence the regularity in BSE. Therefore a comprehensive, continuous and multidimensional programme is developed, aimed at *making BSE a life-long habit*. The programme consists of personal advice, a feedback system with calendars and a link to a breast specialist for those women who detect breat cancer symptoms through regular BSE. No one is left alone with her BSE and everyone knows exactly what to do if breast cancer symptoms occur.

According to many specialists in this field BSE has the basic and primary role in a worldwide fight against breast cancer. Every woman can take advantage of this opportunity. Every decision maker can take advantage of this non-expensive way for the detection of all breast cancers in a country, independent of women's living area.

The Mama Programme can be initiated by decision-makers, medical personnel and women themselves. Women can initiate and go on with the programme themselves on continuous basis. They can also make initiatives to enroll step by step all women in their country.

Mama Programme

Cautious Breast Self-Examination Technique

Inspection

Stand in front of a mirror

a) Is there any retraction of the nipple?

b) Is there any retraction of the skin?

c) Is there a bloody discharge or is the nipple sore?

a), b) and c) should be checked in both the hands-down and the hands-up positions.

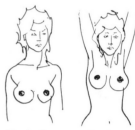

Hands down   Hands up

Palpation

Lie down

d) Are there any lumps in the breasts?

This examination can be accomplished easily by making the skin slippery with soapy water or creme lotion.

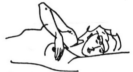

Arm stretched upwards

Use the hand opposite the breast to be examined. Press the breast mildly against the chest sector by sector, using the entire length of the fingers and palm.

Three separate examinations are required for each breast with the arm next to the breast examined in three different positions as shown in the illustrations.

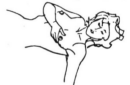

Arm stretched to the side

Benign tumours (non-malignant) are often tender and seem to be harder prior to the onset of menstruation.

Malignant tumours are usually felt as hard lumps, which remain hard between menstruations. They are not always tender when palpated.

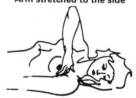

Arm beside chest

Always perform BSE immediately following menstruation. If you no longer menstruate, BSE should still be regularly performed monthly. If you find any breast cancer symptom(s), the breast specialist in your Mama Programme should be contacted immediately.

© G. Gästrin   Almqvist & Wiksell, Uppsala, Sweden 1981

the continuous Mama Programme

Mama Programme

Name _____

Name of key-person_____
(provides information and handles the yearly exchange of "calendars")

Name of breast specialist_____
(to be contacted if you detect breast cancer symptoms)

Calendar for monthly breast self-examination during 19____

(a personal record for you and your breast specialist if required)

Fill in:
- Notes about breast self-examination dates
- Possible breast cancer indications

Right Left	Right Left
January	July ....
February	August ....
March	September ....
April	October ....
May	November ....
June	December ....

If you find any possible breast cancer symptom(s), the breast specialist should be contacted immediately